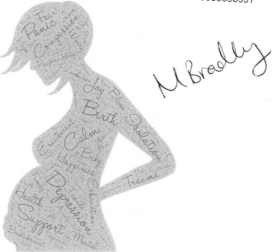

Pangs

Surviving Motherhood and Mental Illness

Michelle Bradley

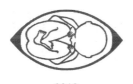

2019

Pangs: Surviving Motherhood and Mental Illness

Michelle Bradley

March 2019

ISBN 978-1-908293-50-3

Published by:

Birthing Awareness

An imprint of CGW Publishing

B 1502

PO Box 15113

Birmingham

B2 2NJ

United Kingdom

www.birthingawareness.com

www.wearepangs.com

Contents

Foreword..4

Introduction..6

PART ONE: WHEN THE WORLD FELL APART............................8

Chapter One - Beginnings..11

Chapter Two - Trust..14

Chapter Three - Rebuilding...18

Chapter Four - Pregnancy No. 1....................................22

Chapter Five - Alexis' Birth..26

Chapter Six - Transitions..38

Chapter Seven - The Turning Point...............................44

Chapter Eight - Rewind Therapy....................................54

Chapter Nine - Loss and Gain.......................................57

Chapter Ten - Cooper's Birth..64

Chapter Eleven - Accidental Baby.................................69

Chapter Twelve - Luna's Birth......................................78

Chapter Thirteen - Back into the Mire...........................84

Chapter Fourteen - Breaking the Stigma........................91

Chapter Fifteen - Changes..97

PART TWO: PERINATAL MENTAL ILLNESS.......................102

Chapter Sixteen - Antenatal and Postnatal Depression......................103

Chapter Seventeen - Antenatal and Postnatal Anxiety Disorder.......107

Chapter Eighteen - Obsessive Compulsive Disorder (OCD)............111

Chapter Nineteen - Birth Trauma/Post Traumatic Stress Disorder.113

Chapter Twenty - Postnatal Psychosis..........................115

PART THREE: TREATMENT...117

Chapter Twenty One - Self Help Techniques..................118

Chapter Twenty Two - Talking Therapies......................130

Chapter Twenty Three - Medication..............................135

Chapter Twenty Four - Physical Wellbeing....................138

Chapter Twenty Five - Social Support...........................144

Chapter Twenty Six - Conclusion..................................147

Resources...153

Acknowledgements..161

Foreword

When I first began to write this book, I was a busy mum of three children under the age of five. In the beginning I thought I was mad to embark on such a project when my schedule and my life were already very full. But this is a story that I need to tell. It is one of how my life was completely taken apart by perinatal mental illness and how I began to put it all back together again, one piece at a time.

Every time I have shared my story at various public speaking events, so many people come up to me afterwards with tears in their eyes to tell me that they have been going through the same thing. It is for them that I decided to put my story to paper. This is for all those women and men who are suffering in silence, afraid to seek help for fear that they will be judged and to those who are reaching out for help and finding it difficult to get what they need.

We need to do better for these parents, particularly our mothers because they are the linchpin of our society, the stitches that hold together the very fabric of our lives. They are where our lives begin and from whom we learn to understand who we are.

If this book makes a difference to one person, to help one person feel a little less lonely and a little more understood, it will have done its job.

To my family, in particular my children, if you are reading this book, before you begin I want you to know that what you will find within these pages will not be a comfortable read. There are aspects of my past that will be difficult to digest. There may be situations and thoughts that I have never shared with you before because I wanted to protect you. There will be times when you may question my feelings for you. I want to tell you this in no uncertain terms - I Love You. I have always loved you and I will always love you. Mental illness is a tricky beast that can make you say, think and feel things that aren't really true. I never want you to question my feelings for you or ever feel that you are to blame for any of the experiences I have had in my life. These events were outside of all of our control and there is no blame and no shame here. We are all survivors. We are all supporters. We are all here, healthy and happy once more and ready to move on. You are my everything and I thank you from the bottom of my heart for your love and support.

Introduction

Before we begin there are a few things you should know. This story is not going to be an altogether happy one. It is the story of how motherhood, in all its wondrous glory can break a person so fully, and how love and support helped to put that broken person back together again.

I will share with you my darkest moments but know from the outset that there is a happy ending. If you have struggled with mental illness, this story may relate to you. You might find yourself triggered by some of the experiences I will share. Be sure to take care of yourself and seek support if you need it.

If you haven't experienced mental illness, I hope that this book may give you an insight into how one of life's most magical moments can turn to darkness and despair. Hopefully it will give you a better understanding and help you to be compassionate towards those who are struggling.

If you are reading this as someone who works with expectant or new parents I have two things I want to say. First of all, thank you for the tireless work you do, particularly those of you who are trying to support parents with very little resources or services in place to assist you. Secondly, it is often difficult to fully grasp the experiences of those you are working with in a short appointment. I hope some of the experiences I share here will give you an idea as to what parents are facing every day and I hope it is helpful to you in your work, in whatever profession that may be.

Stephanie Sparkles said, "I love when people that have been through hell walk out of the flames carrying buckets of water for those still consumed by the fire.

That is what I hope this book will be for you, a bucket of water to help you quench the fire that you, or someone you are supporting, is walking through. As I tell my story, I will also share with you the tools I used to get out of the fire and back to a life I can say with certainty is enjoyable and worth living.

It is my sincerest hope that by sharing this with you that it will, in some way, help break the stigma of mental illness that new parents are facing every day.

This book is split into three parts. In Part One I will share my own experiences of perinatal mental illness, how I recovered and began to help others.

Part Two looks at the types of perinatal mental illness and how you can spot them.

Part Three is a sort of self-help section which will be full of resources, techniques and guidance that you can use yourself in your own recovery, or to support someone who is suffering.

PART ONE:

WHEN THE WORLD FELL APART

Letter to my pre-parent self

Dear pre-parent me,

You are probably reading this in bed. If it's a weekend, it's likely that you will stay there until after midday then roll off the mattress, cook a hot "breakfast" and casually chat with hubby. You might venture into town to shop for something to wear to the pub tonight. You might just stay in your pyjamas all day watching crap TV and eating junk food. Later, you might have sex with your husband. Loud sex. Free sex. You worry about your wobbly tummy but you really have no idea how good you have got it. I wish I was as fat as I thought I was when I was you!

You're also waiting. Waiting for something to happen. For something to begin. You often think about having babies and ache with longing. You also look at other exhausted mums pushing prams and think you don't have the energy for that! You're right. You don't. But I don't think anyone does!

I want to prepare you for the changes that are about to come. Motherhood is everything you expected and more. Those soft skin snuggles, baby gurgles, first steps, first tooth, first word marvels. Your heart will break with love for the little people you are going to bring into the world. You will feel it physically in your gut and not only will you love them with every fibre of your being, you will also feel more loved yourself than you have ever felt in your life. You will crave them when you're not with them. You swear to yourself that you will remember every moment of the wonderful times you have together. You won't. You will forget how they feel and how they smell as they stretch and grow and become more independent from you. You will have a shadow of a memory but it will never be as real nor as tangible. And with all this wonder and awe and love, something else will also come. Something you weren't expecting.

You are about to face the biggest battle of your life and you will almost lose. Anxiety, panic and depression will take you to the darkest of places and tell you that you can't get out. You will look at those sweet babies and feel like you are failing them. You will doubt if you are enough. You will doubt if you will survive. You will have to work so damn hard to pull yourself out of that pit of despair and claw your way back to some sort of normalcy. And when you do it, and you're winning, another baby will come along bringing with it all that wonder and yet once again throwing you into the cycle of panic. And once more you will fight, and you are winning. By the time baby number three makes herself known you will wonder if you can go through it again. You can.

I want you to know that becoming a mother has been the making, the breaking and the reforming of you. "You" as you are now no longer exist. There are no more sleep-ins, no more loud, free, uninhibited sex. In fact, you'll be lucky for five minutes of peace to have a conversation or hold hands, never mind have sex! Plus those wobbly bits are wobblier and accompanied by thick lines of stretch marks, not that you mind too much. Your body is nothing like it was before. Your pelvis still aches, your boobs no longer stand to attention and the wrinkles are setting in. It's not as distressing as you might think so don't worry about it.

Along with your new body, you have a new mind. It's often fraught with anxiety, you snap at the kids when you don't mean to and you are desperate for just half an hour in the day when someone isn't touching you. Until they aren't. Then you want to crawl into bed with those sweet kids and breathe in their scent, feel their soft skin, whisper apologies in their ear and promise to do better tomorrow. You are still figuring this shit out and that's OK. Follow your gut and you will be fine. You will be tested like never before and you will come out the other side. You are scarred but you are strong. Your experiences will open up so many opportunities to help others. You will campaign for better services, you will make a difference to people and your story will have a purpose. You will even find your own passion and start your own business. You are not perfect, but you are enough. And that's all you need to be.

All my love,

Future You x

Chapter One - Beginnings

"Please call an ambulance. I can't breathe, I'm having a heart attack. Oh god please, I need help, I'm dying!"

It was Thursday evening, 9th November to be precise and a day that will stick in my head forever. It was a cold, wet and rainy night and little did I know then, it was the night that was going to change the course of my life forever.

The fire was lit, the room was cosy and snug. The beautiful baby girl I had just given birth to three days earlier was lying tucked up fast asleep in her basket and my husband Eoin was stretched out watching Masterchef.

I was resting on the sofa when out of the blue I was overcome with an intense sensation that I was about to die. My chest suddenly felt tight and I couldn't catch my breath. The room began to spin as I leapt up from my seat, thinking somehow that being upright would prevent me from slipping into oblivion. I began pacing the floor, begging my husband to do something, anything, to help me. I was convinced I was having a heart attack as I struggled for air and shook violently. As my racing pulse pounded in my ears I looked down at my baby girl asleep and blissfully unaware that the sky was falling, and I felt a sickening thud in my the pit of my stomach as I realised that she would grow up without a mother.

This was the beginning of the end of my world for a time and I often look back on that night and wonder, if it hadn't happened how would my life be different?

Before I tell you how that night changed my life, I want to take you briefly back into my past. A journey through my younger years so you can understand how I may have gotten to this point of pacing like a caged animal waiting for my life to end when my daughter's was only just beginning. Like most difficult stories, the problem began in childhood.

I was born in 1984 in Belfast while the civil war (often referred to as 'The Troubles') was still raging on. I am the second-eldest of four children born in a working class neighbourhood right on the border between a Nationalist (Catholic) and Loyalist (Protestant) area. When I think of my childhood I think of the army performing controlled explosions on abandoned cars in front of our house in case they contained bombs. I think of soldiers patrolling the streets and letting us look down the scope of their rifles. I think of marching bands, riots, bomb scares and anger. I think of my dad being forced at gun point up against a wall by a soldier while my three year old brother watched, simply because he was Catholic. I remember, in my six-year old innocence, telling my dad that soldiers weren't all bad, some of them were quite nice actually, and his panicked face telling me never to say that outside of our house.

I also remember playing in the street with my siblings on long summer evenings, sing-alongs with my parents and their friends when they held parties after nights out, dinner at my grandmother's house and late night chats with my sisters. My parents worked hard to make our childhood as happy and as normal as they could given the political turmoil and civil unrest. Despite the frequent controlled explosions, I don't ever remember being worried that a car bomb would actually go off. I never felt afraid for my life or worried for my safety. Even when a family friend was shot dead right beside our house, I never considered that our lives were in danger and that was an incredible feat on the part of my parents.

Of course back then we never knew about trans-generational trauma - the process of trauma being passed down from parent to child through the switching on of certain genes in the body. It never occurred to anybody that the traumas affecting people like my parents and grandparents could ever be transmitted to the next generation simply through their biology. They just worked hard and protected us as best they could. This resulted in a 'pull your socks up' attitude to mental health that has pervaded our society to the very core.

"Life is hard, deal with it."

"Are you feeling sad? Oh well, someone else always has it harder."

"Just get on with it!"

The mothers in our community in those days usually worked. Sectarian discrimination meant that jobs were often hard, manual jobs with low wages. They also raised the babies, cleaned the houses, managed the money, and the men, and the lives of everyone around them. My mother worked a bar job when we were young, spending the day looking after us, cooking, shopping, cleaning and paying the bills before heading out to work as we headed off to bed. Back then communities were more tight knit and you could rely on your neighbours, friends and family - everyone helped everyone else out. We've lost that connection somewhere along the way.

My parents worked hard and they also partied hard. At the weekends we would either stay with our grandparents or a cousin would babysit while they went out and shook off the stresses of the week, often coming home late in the evening with friends for a drink and a sing-song. These are some of my favourite memories as a kid, creeping downstairs to watch them all sing and if I was lucky, someone would give me a pound! It was in these moments that I learned the value of friendship, camaraderie, support and a good sense of humour.

So you see, despite the Troubles and the money worries and the constant unyielding pressure my parents faced, my childhood seems pretty good. But all was not as it seemed.

Chapter Two - Trust

Do you have a secret? I do.

Everyone has secrets, it's a fact of life. Some secrets are small, like 'I fancy the man who delivers the post' or 'I stole a bar of chocolate from the shop once'. Some secrets are big, life-shattering, earth-moving secrets. My secret is one of those.

Despite all the happiness I had in my childhood, there was no way my parents could function under all that pressure without something giving way. I was an outgoing, flamboyant and dramatic child and now that I have children myself, I realise how exhausting that can be. I always craved attention and did everything I could to be different, to stand out and be noticed. With four children to raise and all the pressure that brought, my parents just didn't have the resources needed for an attention-hungry child like myself. Unfortunately that need for attention and to feel special meant that I placed my trust in the wrong person.

I'm not entirely sure when it began but I think I was around six years old when someone close to our family began to take advantage of my need to feel special and used it to his advantage. For the next few years I would be groomed and cajoled into a sexual relationship with this man and for many years afterwards I would believe it had been my idea. I often still question if it was my idea.

As a child I often thought that I was the one doing something terribly wrong and that my abuser needed to be protected. I wouldn't tell anyone, not because he was hurting me but because I didn't want him to be punished for something that was my fault. It was around this time that I began to have nightly panic attacks and anxiety, though I didn't realise then that that was what was happening. I was almost an adult when I discovered that the sick feeling I would get in the pit of my stomach and the racing heart and breathlessness were all symptoms of anxiety.

I remember one day whispering my secret up the chimney because I just needed to get the words out of my body. I remember shortly afterwards I heard the lyrics to a Robson and Jerome song 'I believe that someone in the great somewhere hears every word' and panicking for days waiting to be found out.

The panic meant I couldn't sleep and would wait until everyone was in bed to sneak to the bathroom and read to take my mind off it. If I couldn't go to the bathroom I would lie with a book at my bedroom door and read using the light coming in the crack under the door. There were horrendous nights when there was no light at all. On those nights I would tell myself stories, or lie with no covers on until I was freezing cold to give myself something physical to focus on. I would try to keep my younger sister awake playing word games or recite chapters from books I'd memorised...anything that would stave off the night and the thoughts that would whirl around in my head. I became very angry and confused about what was happening to me and it made me question every relationship that I was a part of. What was normal? What was inappropriate? I struggled to know when a word or a gesture was innocent or suggestive and throughout my life this led to confusing and potentially harmful situations.

I relished the nights when my dad would have a drink and sneak me downstairs to listen to Billy Joel songs with him and I would finally get the attention I craved. I loved these nights because not only was it just the two of us, but because I didn't have to lie in bed submerged in the loneliness of my world of secrets. It made the night so much shorter and the anxiety would ebb away. Looking back I think he was lonely too and needed someone to hear his pain. We became a support to each other. But then day would break, we would both be tired and grumpy, he would be hungover and we would end up fighting. I couldn't comprehend how in the night time he could be so caring and sentimental and in the day time be so cut off and distant, seemingly uncaring at times. I realise now that he had his own demons to battle and it wasn't about me. Still, it made for a tumultuous relationship that we would struggle with for many years.

Flash forward to my teenage years. The sexual abuse had stopped but I still carried with me the weight of my secret, except now it felt different. Over time I had been able to explore what happened to me and move on, but the secret itself remained and I knew that just like that time when I whispered up the chimney, that I would have to say the words out loud to someone to fully allow myself to put it in the past. What I didn't want to do was hurt my family. I had been able to take the experience and use it as a motivation and a force for good. It allowed me to be compassionate towards others and to counsel people who had been through something similar. It gave me a drive to help people, but I also knew that for my family, all it would cause was pain. I was certain they wouldn't be able to see it as anything other than a terrible thing that happened to their daughter, their sister and I didn't see how telling them could help. For many years I would stand outside my parents' bedroom door steadying myself to go and tell them but I couldn't bring myself to. I couldn't see a positive to exposing my secret other than to make myself feel better and that felt incredibly selfish. I held onto the secret , thinking that by shouldering it on my own, I was protecting them from all that pain.

It all came to a head one day after a fight with my mother over cleaning my room. I was nineteen at the time and craved independence and to have some privacy and space of my own. After our row she kicked me out and as I sat on a bus to my aunt's house I was seething with anger. She had called me selfish. How could I be selfish when I was holding this massive burden, just to protect her? At this point in my life I had been secretly going to counselling and as part of my therapy I had written a letter to my abuser explaining in detail what had happened and how it had made me feel. I hid the letter in my bedroom planning to give it to him one day so he would understand what he had done.

After the fight, I messaged my younger sister and asked her to give the letter to my mum so that she would finally know the truth. I was so angry and I couldn't bear to feel so alone for another second. I wanted her to know that I wasn't selfish. I wanted her to understand me, to see me, to get that I wasn't been obstinate or disrespectful by not cleaning my room. I wanted her to know that this seemingly stupid fight was about so much more. It was about my need for privacy and security and safety. I wanted her to know how isolated I felt in my world of secrets and most of all, I was so dog-tired holding this burden, I wanted help. I knew it was now or never but I still feel regret to this day for the way I did it. I was angry and hurt which is never the best head space to be in for a revelation of this magnitude. Still, I can't turn back the clock.

I was petrified that this would be the point when my whole life turned upside down. That this would be the fight to end all fights. That this would be the moment when I would lose everything.

This night changed the dynamics of my family forever.

Chapter Three - Rebuilding

"Sometimes we just need someone to be there for us. Not to fix anything or do anything in particular, simply so that we can feel we are supported and cared for during the hard times."

I arrived on the doorstep of my parents' house later that night and they opened the door with tears streaming down their faces. They bundled me into the tightest hug and we all wept together. I could feel their pain and their anger and I wanted to take it from them. I wanted them to know that I was OK. I wanted to protect them from this horrible thing but I knew I couldn't.

We sat together in our living room while I explained everything that had happened, the years of abuse and how I finally found my voice and said 'No' and that was the end of it. I remember choosing my words very carefully, shielding them from the more difficult details and all the time trying to reassure them that I was fine.

I was so afraid of what they might do next. My mother wanted to call the police but my abuser was dying a slow and painful death of cancer and I didn't see the point. Despite everything that had happened, I still cared for him and felt he had been punished enough. I knew it wouldn't be long until he died and he had children and grandchildren who shouldn't have to bear the weight of what he did, not when they were already dealing with their own grief at his impending passing.

What surprised me more than anything was how my parents really listened to me and took my lead on how to move forward. I was so afraid that the whole situation would spin out of my control and take me down a path I couldn't bear to go down, so to have them respect my wishes and give me their full support was a huge relief. In fact, I truly believe it was the turning point in my relationship with them. They got to understand why I could be so defiant and 'out there' and I began to understand how deeply they loved me and had tried their best for me. We found a new respect and affection for each other and they have been my biggest supporters ever since.

Letting them in on my secret helped us to rebuild as a family and our relationships became solid and strong. This was to be key in helping me overcome my mental illnesses in the future. Understanding each other as we truly were, forgiving each other our shortcomings and striving to be more compassionate towards each other was such an uplifting experience and helped to heal a lot of old wounds. For the first time since I could remember I truly felt like I was part of something, that I wasn't alone on the periphery but part of a team. A team that would have my back from that point on and who would help me grow into a strong, confident and overall happy woman. They helped me lay the foundation on which I would build the rest of my life and an experience which could have easily destroyed any hope for a happy future became a driving force for everything good that happened in my life as an adult.

Around a year before I had finally let go of my secret I had met a boy. A wonderful boy who was to become my husband in years to come and he was the one who convinced me to share my secret with my parents. Without his support, love and backing I would never have had the strength or the bravery to tell my parents the truth. He was then, and is now, my rock and my anchor. With him I felt I could finally just be myself, warts and all and be loved all the same. He made me feel worthy and capable of anything. He has been an integral part of that team who surround me and from whom I draw love and support every day.

The next ten years were some of the happiest of my life. I had found my love, rebuilt my family relationships, I had a great group of friends and I finally settled into my life without this huge weight dragging me down. Having this support network and connection meant that I could begin to open up more about my experiences. Through sharing my story and talking to others, I began to see how many other people had been through similar experiences and I felt this need to gather them all up and fix the broken parts of their lives. I knew there was very little I could do except keep talking and sharing which seemed to give others permission to share their stories and find connection. I didn't realise it then but what I had been unconsciously doing was finding my very own peer support group, surrounding myself with others who understood me on the deepest level and through whom I could better understand myself.

In my late teens I took part in an exchange programme through school and travelled to Denver where I took part in a wonderful programme called BoldLeaders. Through this programme I began to realise my own potential and my ability to create the life I had always wanted. I learned how to be a leader in my own life and in my community for the betterment of all. The life I wanted looked like a strong marriage, a secure home and a football team of babies. I had finally come to a point in my life where everything was as it should be and I was hopeful about the future.

I don't believe life happens by accident. I knew what I wanted from my life and I was determined to get it. Some will say I hen-pecked my husband into marriage when really I just gave him a mighty shove in the right direction! It was the best shove I ever gave. Sixteen years down the line we are as happy and as in love as we've ever been.

But my eye was on the big prize, the one I'd been dreaming of my whole life, the ultimate life experience...parenthood! I was so ready for it.

Six months after we were married, I sat in the bathroom of the recruitment company where I worked and peed on a stick. I sat squirming with excitement as I waited and when I finally saw those two blue lines, I could have burst with excitement. This was it.

Pregnancy. Babies. Motherhood. This is what I had been made for and I was sure that this was the beginning of a fairytale in which I would magically blossom into an earth mother. I would be the picture of patience, grace and love, and raise the most wonderful, well-rounded person in existence. For the first time in my life I felt whole, complete, finished. It was all I had ever wanted and now it was happening. Everything was perfect.

Can you guess the twist yet?

Chapter Four - Pregnancy No. 1

"Your body can stand almost anything. It's your mind you have to convince."

My first pregnancy was, for the most part, everything I thought it would be. I had the standard first trimester morning sickness, the sore hips, nesting! I loved my swelling belly, my softening curves, my thick, lustrous hair. I was in awe that there could be a little person growing inside me and my stomach did a little flip every time I thought of her and I, this little ecosystem working together to make her grow. When I saw her on the screen at our first scan, I laughed and cried so much that the midwife told me off for making the picture jump around while she was trying to take measurements. I was in my element.

My pregnancy was fairly textbook with only a few minor hiccups. One of these being that the baby was measuring small for dates - she turned out to be 8lb 14oz so not small by any comparison! The only other real hiccup I had was first trimester anxiety and even though I had a history of anxiety, I didn't pick up on this warning flag until it was too late.

Some people will say that anxiety in the first trimester is normal and for the most part they are right. Until you hit that magical twelve week mark that everyone tells you about, you are almost holding your breath hoping everything is ticking away as it should. What isn't normal is to have waves of heart-pounding terror and panic attacks. I put it down to hormones and tried to put it out of my mind. You might say I buried my head in the sand.

At some point towards the middle of my second trimester I just 'decided' that I wasn't going to panic any more. I was going to trust my body and my mind to be absolutely fine and I carried on regardless. I practised hypnobirthing, I avoided sugar and caffeine as they were too stimulating. I even lost a lot of weight because I had no appetite, a clear indicator of anxiety for me. I don't know why I didn't see it. I just pottered along pretending it wasn't there and trying not to think about it. The only thing I would acknowledge openly was my biggest fear...panicking in labour.

I spent a lot of my pregnancy thinking about labour and birth. I wasn't afraid of the pain, I honestly did believe that my body was capable of bringing this baby into the world and that I wouldn't need drugs or interventions of any kind. I was, however, preoccupied with the thought of panicking. I was so petrified that I would be in the middle of delivering this baby and would be overcome by that horrific feeling that I was going to die. I knew that if that happened, I would completely lose control and birthing a baby through that seemed absolutely impossible. When I look back at my birth plan I realise I had written it as a design to avoid panic. There has been a lot of talk in the media recently about birth plans with plenty of negative criticism for any woman who should have the nerve to educate herself and prepare for a birth she wants, or should I say, the birth she needs. In fact, Dr. Adam Kay, writes in his "comedic" book This Is Going to Hurt:

"The whole thing was doomed from the start - having a birth plan always strikes me as akin to having a 'what I want the weather to be' plan or a 'winning the lottery' plan. Two centuries of obstetricians have found no way of predicting the course of a labour, but a certain denomination of floaty-dressed mother seems to think she can manage it easily"

I won't even delve in to the misogyny of this quote. I makes me too angry for a measured response but what many health professionals like Dr Kay may fail to understand is that many women like me aren't preparing for a perfect labour and delivery.

We are preparing ourselves mentally for the enormous task ahead and the litany of unknowns facing us when we are at our most vulnerable. These birth plans aren't instruction manuals for a textbook delivery. They are a guide for our carers as to how we need to be spoken with, how we need information presented to us so that we can make the best decisions at the time. They are a signs that scream 'Treat me like a human being. Speak to me with compassion. Understand my terror and my excitement and help me navigate this experience in the best way possible'.

I believe very few women write a birth plan like a checklist of things that must go right. Most understand that there may unexpected circumstances and potentially difficult choices that may take us away from the experience we hope to have. What all birth plans have in common though is that they are the most succinct way of a mother asking to be seen and understood. To be a part of her birthing experience with a semblance of control and not just a body on a bed having things done 'to her' as she performs the most miraculous task there is, bringing forth life. My birth plan was my effort to manage my mental health and had the health professionals who were overseeing my care realised that then perhaps this book wouldn't have needed to be written.

One thing I wasn't prepared for during pregnancy was the antenatal care. I assumed that I would go to my first midwife appointment and someone there would explain what was going to happen over the coming months and what I needed to do. Instead I answered a lot of questions about my medical history, peed into a cup, had some blood drawn and was sent on my merry way. I didn't know when I would write my birth plan, who I would speak to about it, what my options were for where to birth, what was available by way of pain relief. No-one had even heard of hypnobirthing! At each appointment I left feeling like a part on a conveyor belt, just another pregnant lady to be processed and released. I remember towards the end of that pregnancy getting quite bewildered because I wanted to explain my fear of panicking, but it seemed rather pointless given that none of these people would actually be present at my birth!

Looking back with more knowledge and experience, I realise that the health service is missing a key trick here. These antenatal appointments are the perfect place to start asking about mental health. Many women will already be suffering with a mental illness or be in the beginnings of mental illness during their pregnancy. Many women who are diagnosed with postnatal mental illness will have actually been suffering before their babies were born.

Why are we not talking about this? Why are we not taking more time to explain to women that in this key time of their lives where monumental change is happening, that it is OK to talk if you are suffering? Why are we not creating a whole-person wellness plan instead of just a birth plan? We all want healthy babies to be born safely but a healthy baby is not the be-all and end-all, it is the bare minimum! We want healthy babies to be delivered safely to healthy mothers. We need mothers whose mental health is being cared for alongside her physical health. Women are not just vessels through which babies arrive into the world. They are whole human beings with a range of complex emotional and physical needs and we need to start caring for the woman in every way we can. The way a baby arrives into the world is just one part of this picture.

In the next chapter you will read how important it is to care for women emotionally as well as physically and what a huge impact it can have on not just the mother's life but the life of the child and wider family circle. We are failing women by not giving them the appropriate information, care and support during this crucial transition and we need to do better.

So I had spent nine months ignoring the red flags of anxiety and focusing on getting through the birth. I had read all the books, talked through every detail of my birth plan with my husband and we were as prepared as we could possibly be. We just had to wait for her to arrive.

Chapter Five - Alexis' Birth

Birth is one of the most earth-shattering, life-changing experiences a person can go through, whether you are the person giving birth or not. What goes on in the birthing room can affect many things including your physical health, mental well-being, bonding with your baby, relationship to your partner if you have one, and on and on it goes.

On paper, my first birth experience was as straightforward as birth could be. My contractions began at 10.30am on Tuesday 6th November, three days before our due date. What began with niggling period-type pains very soon progressed into full blown, take-your-breath-away contractions.

In the beginning I was very calm. I had been practising hypnobirthing at home and although I was in pain, I was also excited that my baby would soon be here. My only concern was the prevailing worry about panicking in labour. My previous experiences of panic and anxiety had usually circled around my health so being in hospital and in pain was a difficult experience for me.

We went into hospital at 5.10pm and after being examined (4.5 centimetres - woohoo!) I was admitted to the maternity ward to wait for my labour to progress. As I was shown my bed on the ward, the Ward Sister asked my husband to leave and come back at visiting time forty minutes later. What!? This was not the plan! My husband had been prepped to keep me calm and to recognise when I was beginning to spin out of control and bring me back. He knew how unsettling I found hospitals and I was relying on him to get me through this. He couldn't leave me, even if it was only for forty minutes. I couldn't grasp why he couldn't stay with me, especially given that it was only a short time until visiting. But both of us were in a situation we had never been in before, faced with an authority figure we had been raised to respect, and so neither of us stood our ground and off he went to sit in the car park until he was allowed back in.

As I watched him walk down the corridor I could feel my heart beginning to race and I struggled not to cry. I paced the floor and focused on my breathing trying to get back on track, all the while keeping one eye on the clock for 6pm to come around so he could come back in.

My contractions were coming thick and fast by now, lasting two minutes each time and knocking the breath out of me. At that point, I had never felt more vulnerable and alone. There was another woman on the ward who wasn't in labour and I was very conscious of her presence. I didn't want to frighten her with my pain so I did my best to hold it in.

Finally I could bear it no more and I buzzed for assistance. The matronly ward sister came in and I explained that I wasn't getting a break between contractions and asked her to phone my husband. I needed him with me and I was worried he was going to miss the birth. I was assured by the ward sister that as a first time mum, I would be in labour for at least another eight hours and refused to call him. I asked if I could get into a birthing pool but as I wasn't 'far enough along' I was told this wasn't an option and instead she ran me a bath. I'll never understand why I could have a bath but not be in the pool.

The sweet relief of the warm water soothed me and I began to relax and focus on my breathing once again. As she left the room, the ward sister pointed to an orange cord hanging from the ceiling and said "Don't leave it too late to pull that" and walked out. What did that mean? When was I supposed to pull it? What was it for? I couldn't think about it for very long though as another contraction washed over me and I directed all my attention to my breathing.

While I was in the bath the hypnobirthing techniques I had been practising were really helping me stay calm and focused. The aim of hypnobirthing is to focus on staying relaxed. By creating an environment where a woman feels safe, calm and supported the body produces less cortisol (stress hormone) and adrenaline (fight or flight hormone). Both of these hormones interfere with the body's chemical for inducing and progressing labour, oxytocin.

Oxytocin (also known as the love hormone) stimulates contractions and signals the body to deliver a baby. It is also the hormone that is released after a baby is born and placed on the breast to stimulate milk production and encourage bonding. It's the hormone that gives us that feel-good factor when we have sex, kiss our partners or fall in love. Hypnobirthing works with breathing, visualisation and promoting a calm and serene birthing environment to allow for optimum production of oxytocin and lower levels of adrenaline and cortisol.

During pregnancy, any time I felt overwhelmed or stressed, I would listen to the hypnobirthing tracks, close my eyes and allow my body to relax. Practising these skills regularly really helped when it came to labour as I had all these techniques at my disposal without having to think too hard about them and while I was left to my own devices in that bath, I felt calm and confident that things were progressing as they should. As I lay in that bath I was in total control and in tune with my body, listening to my instincts and allowing myself to do whatever I needed to do in order to birth this baby.

By the time my husband arrived back on the ward at 6pm, I was contracting constantly and making a lot of loud mooing noises. I was in a lot of pain but I was managing and felt in total control. I was relaxed and focused, trusting my body's ability to birth this baby. Worried that I seemed to be in a world of my own, my husband called a midwife, telling her that I was making 'a lot of weird noises'. When the midwives came in to examine me I had gone from 5cm dilated to 10cm dilated in less than forty minutes. I fully credit this to the hypnobirthing and my ability to get myself into a calm and relaxed state. All that oxytocin was just flooding my body, just as it should.

This is where it began to go wrong.

My midwife asked me to get out of the bath so we could move to labour ward but I couldn't bring myself to get up. In between each contraction I was asked to stand up, but the gap between contractions was so short that before I even made a move to stand, another one washed over me and I had to lay back down. I didn't understand why I needed to move. Things were going well, why couldn't I give birth here?

Every time they asked me to move I got more and more stressed out. I could feel the panic rising in my chest and I begged them to just leave me alone. Eventually two midwives grabbed me under each arm, hoisted me up and sat me in a wheelchair. A gown was hurriedly thrown over me and I was wheeled through the maternity ward at visiting hour, with all the new daddies watching me half naked and moaning with pain. Ground swallow me up! And if I thought the contractions were painful in the bath, they ramped up tenfold sitting in that wheelchair. I'm sure the stress didn't help!

Down in the labour ward I was wheeled into a delivery room and helped onto a bed. I didn't want to be lying down, I wanted to be upright or in water. I asked to get in the birthing pool and the midwives seemed a bit put out, telling me it would take half an hour to fill. I remember their hesitant glances to each other and I realised that they didn't seem confident assisting with water births. They would much rather have had me on my back so they could see what was going on. I insisted on the birthing pool and finally, as I lowered myself into the water I felt myself begin to unwind. The move from the maternity ward bath down to labour ward had been a such jarring experience and I knew I needed to get back in the zone to boost my oxytocin levels and get things back on track.

I was barely in the pool though when my midwives asked me why I wasn't pushing. I told them I didn't feel like pushing. My contractions had gone from being strong and regular to patchy and varying in intensity. They explained that as I was ten centimetres dilated, I only had two hours to get this baby out before they would need to intervene. Immediately my attention was now on the clock on the wall. I pushed and pushed and pushed for what seemed like an eternity, each time my contractions would seem to falter halfway through and lose momentum.

I was so stressed and out of my mind with worry that I started to doubt if I could actually do this. The only thing that stopped me from progressing to a full blown panic was the gas and air. It took the edge off the pain and made me feel pleasantly detached from the intense environment I now found myself in. Until they took it away. They said I was 'abusing it'. And so the one thing that was giving me some sort of comfort was stripped away and I found myself reeling with breathlessness, panic and despair.

This wasn't helped when every time I looked at my midwives faces they seemed either concerned or annoyed so I clamped my eyes shut and refused to acknowledge they were in the room. This was difficult though as they repeatedly told me to stop making noise as if I could help it.

"Focus your energy down into pushing, not into vocalising".

I was going to focus my energy into kicking one of them in the head if they didn't leave me alone! They told me to 'push on, push on, push on' repeatedly even when I had no urge to push. There was one midwife in particular who lacked any sign of compassion and seemed bored and frustrated with me. She made me feel like I was making a terrible fuss over nothing. Her 'push on' translated in my head to 'You're not doing this well enough. You're terrible at giving birth. You are so shit at this'. I was in the middle of the most exhausting and unyielding experience of my life and the people who were supposed to be my cheerleaders became my tormentors.

At one point I opened my eyes, looked right into Eoin's and asked him to help me. He just told me to do what the midwives said. He had given up on the hypnobirthing. All the techniques we had worked on together, the techniques that were working so well a few hours before had been forgotten and once again I felt totally alone. I could see he was concerned and felt more comfortable letting the professionals take the lead, trusting them to get us through this. I don't blame him. It was an overwhelming experience for him too and one that he felt totally helpless in. Before we went into labour, I told him that I would try very hard not to be the stereotypical ranting wife, raging at the husband for getting her in this position. I was very aware that there were two of us in this situation and that this birth wasn't just mine alone. As I asked him to help me, I'm sure he would have moved heaven and earth if he could to make it easier for me but it was as much out of his control as it was out of mine at that point.

Two hours of pushing later and time was up. I was once again forced out of the water and made to walk dripping wet down a corridor and back into the bed I'd been assigned earlier - the last place I wanted to be. Immediately there was a change in the atmosphere. The midwives had gone from being critical, nervous bystanders to being engaged and energetic. They had me where they wanted me. Where they felt comfortable.

I was no longer a part of this birthing process as they took over to do the 'necessary' to get my baby out. They paged an obstetrician who was on his way. While they waited, one of them said,

"Mrs Bradley, I'm just going to give you a wee epi."

I had no idea what that meant until moments later I felt her cutting me. I wasn't given an option to consent or refuse, so short was the time between the statement and the cutting. If she had bothered to read my birth notes she would also have known that given my history of sexual abuse, having things done to my body without my consent was a big trigger. I wonder if Dr Kay attributes any of the failures of his patients birth plans to the health professionals making it so?

She told me to push again and try as I might I couldn't get that baby out. She then asked me to look down towards her where, to my horror she was holding up a mirror to my swollen, bruised and bloody vagina to tell me that that flash of black hair I could see was my baby's head! She probably thought this would motivate me to push. She didn't consider that the sight of how damaged and gruesome my body looked might kick off a panic. She didn't read my hospital notes where it was clearly stated that I had health anxiety and found it very distressing to experience bodily sensations or changes that were outside the norm. I threw my head back and cried at the pain, the damage and the crushing fear that I couldn't do this. I was either going to die, or kill my baby because I couldn't get her out on my own.

Moments later a handsome doctor arrived, rolled up his sleeves and explained to me that he was just going to pop a suction cap onto my baby's head and deliver her 'for me'. What a guy. What a hero. I was 'allowed' gas and air again for this part as he cut me again (without consent) and on he went, doing the job that I couldn't do.

I bore down as her head was delivered and suddenly, without warning my knees were shoved up to my chest. I discovered later when going through my birth notes that he had called this a 'prophylactic McRoberts manoeuvre' to prevent shoulder dystocia as my baby's head hadn't turned when she was born. The midwife taking me through my notes told me that she felt this was completely unnecessary. It also led to further tearing which required quite a number of stitches, not to mention the fact that my body was being 'managed' without any explanation or even eye contact. I was once again in a position where I had no control over my body and was at the mercy of a man who could seemingly do as he pleased. I understand that this man was there to help me and I know that this wasn't the same situation as the abuse I had been through as a child, however, being in this weak and submissive position was a massive trigger and all it would have taken was a conversation, an explanation, my consent or some sense that I had some say in what was happening to me to make this situation much more bearable.

Another pull of the suction cup later and my baby was born and whisked away to be checked over. I didn't even get a look at her. I felt a huge wave of relief wash over me that it was finally over. Relief and exhaustion. I puffed on the gas and air while the doctor stitched me up, even managing in my drunken haze to flirt with him a little (he was very handsome!). The respite didn't last long though. The doctor made a joke about how I had made a mess of his 'nice clean floor' with all the blood. I immediately began to panic. Was I bleeding to death? Was I OK? I didn't say any of this out loud. I didn't trust him to be honest with me so I just lay back with tears rolling down my cheeks praying that I wouldn't die. I sucked on the gas and air as Dr. Hero stitched me up and I floated out of the room where the panic couldn't get me.

I remember in my haze asking if the baby was OK. I didn't ask because I was particularly interested but because I felt it was something I should probably ask. That's what mothers do right? Show concern for their children? Looking back, that was the first sign that things weren't right. I used to remember that moment with the most horrendous guilt but now I know that it wasn't my fault that my mothering instinct hadn't switched on. I had just been through an ordeal, I was exhausted, emotionally drained and just needed some time to get back to feeling safe and secure. I was worried about my own health. My body felt alien to me and I found it incredibly distressing. I didn't feel like I had done something amazing, or that I had done anything at all. I felt like things had been done to me. That my body belonged to others, just like it had all those years ago and I had no say in what happened. I was reduced to a whimpering child submitting to the will of adults in positions of authority. All my mental resources were redirected to survival mode and I hadn't the capacity to feel anything other than my self-preservation instinct.

The most infuriating thing about the entire labour and delivery is that, had I been left alone to just get on with it, if I hadn't been coaxed and cajoled to push for hours on end when my body was clearly not ready to birth this child, I have no doubt that I could have birthed her without any problem. This 'failure' wasn't mine. It was the health professionals who didn't read my notes, didn't show any compassion and treated me like a piece of meat on a slab.

Shortly afterwards, Eoin and I were left alone with this little baby. He sat cuddling her while I just lay in a state of shock. He kept telling me I needed to hold her but I couldn't even lift my arms. I wasn't interested in holding her. I just wanted her to be somewhere else for a while until I got myself back on an even keel. I couldn't face the fact that I was now a mother to someone when I felt like such a child myself. It was too much.

Before she was born I had made the decision to breastfeed. I wanted to give her the best start in life and I liked the idea of my body continuing to help her grow and develop. I could hear her in her daddy's arms making little sucking sounds and rooting around for me. Eventually I did take her and she latched onto my breast for her first feed. I felt nothing. She was a squishy, pink stranger and I felt no connection whatsoever. All the bonding and love I had felt for her in the womb seemed to belong to someone else. To an imaginary baby who hadn't yet materialised. What was wrong with me?

The midwives came in to check we were all okay and told Eoin that he needed to go home. Once again I begged them to let him stay. I needed him there to comfort me, to talk to me and help me find my equilibrium. I was petrified of staying in hospital as a rule and after what I had just been through, I couldn't fathom the thought of being left alone with this baby and no support. Needless to say, my trust in the midwives to support me was severely lacking. He was told in no uncertain terms that he had to leave and he could come back tomorrow afternoon. I sobbed as he left and felt this crushing weight of responsibility for this child. How could I care for her when I felt so vulnerable and needy myself? For the third time that night, I felt utterly alone.

I was taken up to the maternity ward where I was left alone for the remainder of the night, unable to sleep, just staring at this baby and wondering what the fuck had just happened to me. It didn't help that my phone had died so I couldn't text Eoin for help and support. A few weeks earlier I had been to the maternity ward for monitoring and had left my charger there. I asked the midwives if I could have it back so I could get in touch with my husband. Four times I asked that night and it never materialised. I was totally cut off.

Every time the baby needed to be fed or changed, I struggled out of the bed to lift her, and then not being able to use my arms to ease myself back on to the bed because I was holding her, I just had to fall over onto the mattress and work my way up to a sitting position slowly and painfully. When I buzzed for help, it didn't come or it came too late. It was just me and her trying to figure it out on our own.

Did I love her then? I don't know. I was in awe of her. I couldn't stop looking at her brown eyes and tiny fingers and the smell of the top of the head was intoxicating, but I didn't feel love like I had felt it for my husband. There were no butterflies, no rush of undeniable 'mother love'. That did come in time but in the beginning, its absence was as solid as the walls around me.

What was wrong with me? This was everything I had ever wanted. Here I was with this perfect little human in my arms who was so wanted and so longed for and all I felt was, what? Curiosity? I felt so ungrateful and ashamed of myself, something it took a long time and a lot of work to forgive myself for.

The next morning after a night of no sleep, a very kind midwife came to check how I was. She asked about the birth but I just shook my head and said,

"Well, she made it through OK".

She then went through a checklist, asking me different questions about my health.

"How is your bleeding?"

"I have no idea, how should it be?"

"Do you have any pain in your legs?"

"I have pain all over."

I remember the ridiculousness of telling her my big toe was excruciatingly sore and asking if that something to worry about.

How had we got to the 21st century and still no one was talking about how you should feel after birth? How was I expected to tell a midwife if my stitches were healing normally when I had never had my vagina stitched before? How was I supposed to know all this stuff when nobody had told me what it was I was supposed to know?

I asked to be discharged as quickly as possible. I couldn't stay in that place one more hour with the crying babies, the inescapable heat, the grey tea and soggy lunch. My husband finally arrived to take us home and I'd never been so relieved to see anyone in my life. As I hobbled out of the maternity ward I gave them all an imaginary middle finger and a mental "Fuck you".

With the birth of my daughter came the death of the person I thought I was. It was the beginning of a long spiral down into a darkness that would threaten my very existence. Was my birth experience the reason I suffered with postnatal mental illness? I won't credit it with the entire blame but it played a huge part in what was to happen next. I had walked into that hospital feeling prepared, in control and ready for what was to happen. I left feeling violated, worthless and incapable. No parent should have to start their journey that way. To leave a hospital responsible for a tiny human and to feel as shaken and as incompetent as you have ever felt in your life is a horrendous position to be in.

Some will say that my birth may have left me feeling that way regardless. Maybe I was naive going into it and I'm being too harsh on the midwives. They may be partly right, I may have been naive. But even if that was the case, my birth experience would have been helped by several things.

Firstly, compassion from the women who were supposed to be caring for me. I understand that their job is to make sure the baby is born healthy and safe. That is the bare minimum of their job, but they cannot separate the needs of the mother from the needs of the child. The mother and the child are one and need to be treated as such. It doesn't take an awful lot to be kind and encouraging. To ask permission before cutting someone. To take a moment to read the birth notes and understand the woman you are caring for in all her complexity. We are not simply vessels in which to carry babies. A little bit of understanding and tact can go a long way. The way a woman is spoken to will determine whether she feels empowered and part of her birth experience, or disregarded and useless.

Secondly, the health professionals need to recognise and acknowledge their own hang ups. The midwives assigned to me were not comfortable with water births. They didn't know how to tell when my waters had broken when I was in the pool. From the moment I asked for the pool, they were actively trying to get me back onto a bed. Their need to feel comfortable impacted everything about my labour and put obstacles in my way that didn't need to be there.

I also discovered after the birth that when they told me to begin pushing and put me on that two hour clock, my baby's head hadn't descended enough for me to push. I spent all that time exhausting myself and distressing my baby when my body wasn't ready. I believe this two hour time limit was to get me out of the pool and back into the midwives' comfort zone.

And finally, don't assume that because you are in a position of authority, that you have the right to ignore the wishes of a patient and do unto them as you see fit when they are at their most vulnerable. Involve women in their care. Explain the benefits and the risks of everything and trust them to make the decision that is right for them, even if that decision makes you uncomfortable. Believe it or not, mothers want their babies to be born safely too and will not go out of their way to object to an intervention if it is in their best interests. But the decision is THEIRS. Not yours.

The care I received during my first birth experience was such that when I left that hospital I wanted to curl up in a ball and forget that I had ever even had a baby. I wanted to rewind and undo everything so that I could feel like myself again and not this weak and pathetic thing I felt I had become.

And that was only the beginning.

Chapter Six - Transitions

For three days after my daughter's birth, I didn't sleep. Not. One. Wink. I don't know why I didn't sleep, I think I was still in a state of shock. I would lie in bed in the darkness of those winter nights and replay her birth over and over and over again in my head. Why did they do this? Why didn't I say that? Why didn't it go differently? Why am I still thinking about this!?

Every time I looked at my daughter it was in complete wonderment that she was here and that I had made her. She seemed so amazing to me but I didn't feel that pang of love in my chest. I remember the day after she was born saying to my husband "I'd die for her but I just don't think I love her enough". In my head I thought I didn't love her at all. The statement seems so silly to me now when I look into her big, brown eyes and my love for her hits me right in the gut. But it was so true to me then that I wondered what was wrong with me.

I also spent those first few days obsessing over the state of my body. Was this bleeding normal? Was this pain normal? How will I know if I need to seek help? This was the beginning of the most severe health anxiety I had ever experienced and it would grip me for the next several years. Every time the midwife called to the house I got her to check my stitches for signs of infection, an indignity in itself, lying on the sofa naked from the waist down and with one leg up in the air! I would wait nervously as she took my blood pressure to see if it was within normal range. I didn't understand why no-one had explained how I would feel after birth and wondered if every little twinge was normal. I felt like I had been hit by a bus! Why did nobody prepare me for that? The pain and bleeding lasted for almost two months, during which time I couldn't walk for long stretches before feeling like my vagina was going to fall off! I couldn't drive my car so I spent most days on the sofa, trapped in my house. But that wasn't even the worst part.

Three days after the baby was born (we named her Alexis but for almost a year I almost always just called her 'the baby'), I went into total meltdown. It began in the early evening as we lay watching TV. The baby was asleep in her moses basket and I was curled up in the fetal position on the sofa, the only position that didn't result in nauseating pain. I was suddenly overcome with a wave of heat and dizziness and in my already heightened state of alert, my brain completely overreacted and sent me into a massive panic.

I jumped up off the sofa and started pacing the floor struggling to breathe. I grabbed my discharge notes and started furiously flicking through the pages of advice for what to do if you can't breathe and your heart feels like it's about to explode. I began to cry and begged my husband to call an ambulance. I'm quite lucky that my husband had witnessed me in a state of panic before and recognised it for what it was. He tried to hold me but I couldn't sit still and didn't want to be confined. I walked out the front door in my pyjamas and began pacing up and down the street trying to settle myself.

Wave after wave of panic crashed down on me for the next four hours as I switched from feeling keyed up and unable to stop moving, to feeling like I was about to pass out with exhaustion. I called my mum in a total state, babbling on about feeling like I was dying and frantic for her to help. She came over right away and set about trying to distract me from the panic. She made me get out my breast pump which was still in the box and got me to sit and read the instructions so I could express some milk. This would allow for Eoin to feed the baby while I got some rest. She blamed this feeling on breastfeeding and thought I was putting too much pressure on myself. I tried to explain that the baby and the breastfeeding weren't the problem. I wasn't panicking about the baby, she was fine. I was afraid that I was going to die. Either way, the process of sorting out the breast pump gave me a focus and helped to reduce the terror as I slowly began to calm down.

Finally I crashed on the sofa and closed my eyes but even then I couldn't sleep, worried that my mum would leave or that I would die in my sleep. I closed my eyes and pretended to be asleep and just listened to the TV and my mum and husband talking. I was also consumed by the thought of walking up the stairs to go bed. This was a strange thing to be worried about but it consumed me over the coming months. Every evening after dinner I would think about the process of walking upstairs to go bed and the thought of lying awake in the dark and the silence petrified me. I didn't understand why. Maybe the silence meant my thoughts could run riot. Maybe the dark allowed images of my daughter's birth to burst forth in full technicolour. Maybe it was my mistrust in my own body, constantly afraid that the minute I let my guard down my heart would stop or my brain would just cease to function. On many occasions as I began to fall asleep, I would be sharply awoken by a buzzing sensation in my head that felt like my brain was vibrating. Every time it would jolt me awake and I would be hit with a panic attack, worried that I had a tumour or an aneurysm. Often-times I would also be just on the cusp of sleep and would feel as though I had no air in my lungs and couldn't breathe. I would jump up gasping for air, taking big deep breaths and trying to prove to myself that my lungs were actually working.

This disruption to my nights only led to more difficult and dark days. I would usually wake in the morning with a feeling of dread in the pit of my stomach as though I were about to attend a job interview I hadn't prepared for. And that's what parenthood is right? The world's toughest job interview where you spend every day winging it and hoping you're doing a good job? When the day starts with this fear and your sleep has been disturbed by both your own body and your baby waking to be fed, needless to say trying to do all the things that could potentially make you feel better seems impossible.

I knew that eating better would help but I could barely make myself toast never mind a healthy balanced breakfast. When I say I couldn't make toast, at this point in my life this was literally true. In those early weeks of terror the thought of doing anything other than lying on the sofa filled me with complete panic. To try and combat this I set myself three small goals every day, knowing that if I could accomplish those I would feel more confident. The aim was to gradually increase the difficulty of these goals until I felt I could cope. The first day that I set these goals, number one on the list was to make myself tea and toast. Up until that point I had been paralysed either in bed or on the sofa, petrified to stand up because I felt so shaky and dizzy, and with the completely irrational thought running round my head that if I stood up I would either die or completely lose my shit. By sitting still I felt safe.

So I challenged myself to get up and make myself toast. I remember the look on my husband's face as I talked out loud to myself, willing myself to stand up, spending half an hour in self-conversation trying to convince myself that this wasn't a big deal, it was just toast right!? When I finally got up I was crying uncontrollably and shuffled slowly into the kitchen waiting for the moment when I would drop dead. My hands trembled as I took the bread out of the packet and I dropped it more than once trying to get it in the toaster. The few minutes it took the bread to toast were interminable and I spent them bent over double, trying to catch my breath and battling with stomach-churning nausea. When the toaster popped I almost jumped out of my skin. I took it back to the living room where I wept so hard with relief and confusion that I couldn't actually eat it. Why was this so fucking hard? How could I look after a baby when I couldn't even make toast? What the fuck was I going to do?

That is the nature of anxiety though. It will fill your brain completely with irrational thoughts and make the smallest task seem like climbing Everest. It will erode your self-confidence and make you feel more weak and vulnerable than you have ever felt in your life. For that to happen when you have just had a new baby and are supposed to be relishing motherhood seems more cruel to me than anything I've ever experienced.

The other problem with anxiety is that when it is left untreated and unmanaged for too long, it begins to erode any sense of hope and opens the door for depression to creep in. That's where I found myself when my daughter was four months old.

We were at home late one evening, the baby sleeping soundly in her cot. We had just got into bed when I was taken over by yet another panic attack, a particularly bad one. I tried my best to get it under control but it just kept washing over me again and again until I could bear it no longer. I got dressed, lifted the baby out of her cot and put her into the pram and asked my husband to come on a walk with me. I felt so trapped and claustrophobic indoors, I just needed to be out in the open in the fresh air. I say fresh, it was the depths of winter and the weather was atrocious.

We walked and walked around our neighbourhood, with me sobbing all the while and generally looking like I had lost my mind. Eoin listened patiently as I rehashed my birth experience for the thousandth time and poring over the last few months of anxiety which had gotten completely out of control. I had been obsessed with getting sick to the point that I overcooked our dinners so we didn't get food poisoning. I held my breath as I passed people in the street in case they had germs. I visited the doctor with a hand written list of things I thought were wrong with me and asked for tests. I spent my days walking around town so that if I suddenly collapsed, there would be people around to help my baby.

Anxiety controlled my every thought, my every movement. I consciously took each stair at a time in case I tripped and fell with the baby. If Eoin was five minutes late in from work, I had horrible 'daymares' imagining him crushed in a car wreck. My body wasn't to be trusted either, with every twinge, every pain, every strange sensation blown out of all proportion to the point where I was just waiting around for the inevitable heart attack to take me.

On that night when we went walking, I was at absolute breaking point. All I could see stretched out in front of me were years of dark, grim and difficult times. Everything seemed so bleak, it was like all the colour had gone from the world. My pervading thought was that the world was impossibly cruel and I had brought a baby into this hell. I felt so selfish for bringing her into the world for her to suffer like I was suffering and I wanted to rewind the clock and forget about having children altogether.

I could imagine her at my age, going through this horrendous ordeal and nothing was more painful to me than thinking that my precious baby would ever have to go through what I was going through. I couldn't see a future where there was anything but pain and suffering. It was that night that I wept to my husband that I really didn't want to die but that I couldn't go on much longer living this hell and if I had a gun or a pill I would put myself out of my misery. The only thing that kept me clinging to life was the pain that my death would cause to my family. That night was a turning point for all of us.

Chapter Seven - The Turning Point

The next morning I found myself in my doctor's surgery at an emergency appointment made by my husband. He told me it was time to see a doctor and that I couldn't manage this alone any more. I knew he was right but I still felt like a failure as a mother. Motherhood was all I had ever wanted. I had always been so on top of things before she was born. I was confident and self-assured even through my previous mental health struggles. I felt like I was letting my baby down and that I just wasn't good enough for her. As I sat in the waiting room, I tried to practise what I was going to say to the doctor. She needed to know how serious it was without making it sound serious enough for her to phone social services. I had this image of a social worker arriving at my door to confirm what I already thought I knew, that I wasn't fit to be a mother and that my daughter would be better off with someone else. I was torn between needing help and not wanting to ask for help. I was ashamed that I wasn't coping and to find myself in the doctor's surgery was validation that I was failing everyone so completely, most of all my baby girl.

When we were finally called, I sat down facing my really lovely G.P. and began to cry. Everything I had rehearsed went out the window as the months of suffering poured out of me in a barely comprehensible babble while snot and tears streamed down my face.

"I think I have postnatal depression" I wept as I described the crippling panic and anxiety, this sense of hopelessness and thoughts of suicide. I couldn't look at her face as I spoke, instead I focused on picking at the cuticles around my finger nails making them bleed in the process. When I finally finished I waited with baited breath for her to declare me insane and insist on removing my baby from my care.

"Right," she said leaning forward and taking control of the situation, "first of all, you don't have postnatal depression. You have generalised anxiety disorder and we can treat that very easily".

My GP is one of those women who seems to always have a plan of action and she immediately set about trying to 'fix' me. She explained about beta blockers and how they stop your heart reacting to adrenaline, which makes anxiety easier to manage.

"Surgeons take these before surgery. They're out of your system in twelve hours and you can take them while you're breastfeeding".

It sounded like the perfect solution but it wasn't going to work for me. I tried to explain that my health anxiety meant that any potential side effects from the medication were going to send me over the edge and I was already so vulnerable that I couldn't risk getting worse.

"Try them for seven days and if they don't work, come back to me".

I spent the next seven days staring at those pills and never taking one. Several times I raised one to my mouth and shaking, set it back down again. I halved them, then quartered them, and still couldn't bring myself to swallow one.

My GP had all the best intentions but she missed one crucial thing. In her need to 'cure' me she forgot to listen to me. I came away feeling more hopeless than before because I had asked for help, and the help I received wasn't going to work. After seven days I went back and tried to explain again. This time she gave me a lower dose of the beta blockers to minimise the side effects and signed me up for cognitive behavioural therapy, or CBT as it's commonly known. Why wasn't I offered CBT in the first instance?

How many women just went away and took the pills, not realising that there were other options? From my many conversations with women going through perinatal mental illness, I have found that the standard response to asking for help is to be given pills and sent away. It is in exceptional cases that women are offered any kind of talking therapy as a first response, or even a combination of medication and therapy which has been proven to be the most effective treatment. While medication can and does reduce the severity of anxiety and depression, it doesn't get to the root cause. It manages the symptoms but doesn't cure the disease. What we need is a multi-disciplinary approach to mental illness, to treat the whole person with a range of resources to increase the likelihood of full recovery. Needless to say, I was one of the 'lucky' ones in that my GP was at least providing CBT as an option.

CBT is a type of therapy that addresses how your brain processes thoughts, emotions and sensations, giving you tools to take control of your thought processes and thus reducing anxiety and panic. It is best given intensively for a few months, at least once a week. My GP could only offer me thirty minutes, once a month for a maximum of six sessions, with a qualified CBT therapist. It wasn't nearly enough but I did find the sessions I had very helpful. I began to understand how my fight-or-flight response was on constant alert and learned techniques to help rationalise my thoughts and calm my nervous system. The panic attacks lessened in severity though I was still suffering anxiety on a daily basis. It seemed more manageable though and got me out of my crisis state. While I wasn't anywhere near recovered, at least I could control the anxiety a little better.

When I finished my CBT sessions, I didn't feel that I could go back to my GP for more help. It seemed to me that the only resources they had at their disposal were those I had already availed of (medication and CBT) and so I didn't think they could help me any more than they already had. I wasn't sure what exactly I needed but I knew I wouldn't find it there.

Frustrated at not being able to identify and access what help I needed I finally began to get angry and this was when things began to change. I was so distressed all the time, and I could see myself losing this precious time with my baby. Then I found some fight. I began to research postnatal anxiety and depression, and to seek therapies privately, and crucially I began to find people who were going through the same thing.

I should say at this point that throughout this tumultuous time, my family (both immediate and extended) were such a huge support to me and I don't know how I would have gotten through this illness without them. Often-times, I would drive to my parents' house or meet with my sisters and be in a state of inconsolable torment. Just being near them, having a cup of tea and sharing how I was feeling was usually enough to help me settle myself. I'm sure on many occasions they would have liked nothing less than to hear me once again rehash what I was going through, but they were patient with me all the same.

I remember explaining how I was feeling to my mother-in-law and would watch her eyes fill with tears at my distress. She wanted nothing more than to help me feel better and it was in these moments that I realised that I wasn't alone. My family stood behind me, reminding me constantly that I could get through this and holding me up when I didn't feel like I could stand on my own. It takes a lot of inner strength to support someone through a mental illness, particularly if you have never experienced it yourself and find it hard to understand. It's so difficult to just 'be' with the person without trying to fix them, but that is often all a person needs, for you to be present. My family were present for me and I will never forget it.

It was shortly after Alexis' first birthday when I really began to search in earnest for help and support outside of my family unit. I began to look for the people who were like me. As amazing as my family had been, I really needed to talk to people who had been through what I had been through, in particular people who had recovered and who could give me hope. In my naivete I assumed that a quick Google search would bring up a list of groups in my area that I could attend and meet people who were going through the same thing. Boy was I wrong! Not only could I not find any face to face support groups, in this age of social media I couldn't even find an online group for people in my country.

For a while I sat despondent, worried that maybe I was the only one who felt this way. Maybe everyone else was just 'getting on with it' and I was the only one who was stuck. It took me some time to realise that maybe, just maybe, there were people like me looking for the same thing and not finding it. Maybe there were others feeling like they were the only ones. At the time I had been listening to a podcast and the phrase 'If not me, who? If not now, when?' was repeated often. It came to my mind at that moment and I thought "Why not me? Why don't I start a support group?" I decided then to set up an online peer support group called PANGS NI. I imagined that it would just be me in the group posting comments to myself and proving that I was, in fact, the oddball who couldn't quite get a handle on this motherhood thing. Two days later, I had forty four members. As I write this book I have nearly five hundred! One mum captured this perfectly when she wrote:

"This is obviously something a lot of us were just waiting for."

It was in turns a relief to know I wasn't alone, and an eye-opener into how many people were actually struggling and not getting the help they needed. The group was full of stories of women who were desperately searching for help and hitting brick walls. GPs were routinely offering anti-depressants as the only solution and the waiting list for talking therapies was so long that it left many families in limbo, wanting to get out of this dark place they were in and having no one to guide them. Women who were suffering with antenatal depression and anxiety were having a particularly hard time as the waiting list for therapy was usually nine months or longer, by which stage their pregnancies would be over and they would be in the midst of surviving life with a newborn and mental illness.

At the time of writing this book, 80% of women in Northern Ireland have no access to specialist services for their mental health during and after pregnancy. There is no mother and baby unit on the island of Ireland meaning that those women who require hospitalisation for their mental health are separated from their babies and placed on general psychiatric wards, thus compounding the problem. Women whose illness registers as mild to moderate in severity often get no help whatsoever, despite suffering daily and for long periods of time.

There is a perinatal psychology team based in Belfast and made up of one psychiatrist and one psychologist. They can only see women who have birthed there and even then, if you are not an in-patient or pregnant you can't access the service and are instead referred to the waiting list for the Adult Mental Health team. As the Adult Mental Health teams cover all mental illness, not just perinatal, needless to say the waiting lists are long.

Northern Ireland is by no means alone in this. Around the world, women and their families are suffering needlessly with mental health issues, and the effects are wide-ranging. A recent study on Adverse Childhood Experiences reports that having a parent with a mental illness is a key indicator for difficulties later in life, with the child's own mental and physical health being put at risk. During pregnancy, mental illness in the mother is shown to switch on those genes in the baby that make them prone to mental illness later in life.

When we take all that into consideration, along with the fact that parents are carrying out the most important job of all - raising the future of our species - why is it that we don't invest in the health and wellbeing of our parents? Why is this role so undervalued? Where are the support systems parents need to fulfil this role without having to sacrifice their own mental and physical health? We are getting it so wrong.

PANGS NI was a real life-line for me while I was in the midst of my own struggle. It was, and still is, a place to share my darkest thoughts, my deepest worries and my most irrational fears with people that I know understand me. The women in the group have been there for me many times in the middle of the night, when I was in the full throes of a panic attack and needed someone to talk too. My husband would be asleep and I didn't want to constantly disturb him so I would go onto the group, get all my scary thoughts out of my head and almost always there was someone else there to help me through it. Sometimes that was all I needed, to get the thoughts out. It was at times like that when I couldn't phone my GP or my counsellor but I needed to be heard, to be seen and understood. PANGS NI gave me that. And in return, as my struggle got a little easier I was able to give hope to those coming behind me, to share the tools and techniques that I found helpful and make someone else's load a bit lighter.

It also provided some respite for my husband and my family. Around the time I started PANGS NI, I had been rehashing my birth and postnatal experiences to my family for over year. They tried their best to support me but there was only so much they could do and only so often they could listen to the same stuff over and over again without getting frustrated themselves. To say my marriage suffered would be an understatement. At times my husband was effectively my carer, having to work from home regularly when I couldn't bear to be alone with the baby, forcing me to eat when anxiety robbed me of my appetite and spending every other moment listening to me recycle the same conversation about how I was feeling. We no longer did anything fun together. We used to enjoy going out for meals but I was so worried about food poisoning that we stopped going, or we would go to a restaurant, eat and then spend the remainder of the evening working through a panic attack at the thought of getting sick. I didn't find any enjoyment in any of the things we used to do so we often spent our evenings doing nothing. Sex was last on my list of priorities and so the intimacy we had went right out the window. There were many nights were we sat side by side on the sofa, not speaking or touching, both drained and unable to find the energy to work on our relationship. I waited for the day when he would finally just give up and leave me. After all, the woman he fell in love with wasn't here any more. She had been replaced by this trembling mess who couldn't function on even the most basic level. I would often wake from a dream in which he had walked out on me and reel for hours, unable to look at him, the feeling of hurt very real and very possible. To be able to relieve him of some of the pressures of having a wife with a mental illness played a big part in preventing our marriage from totally breaking down. Having somewhere else to express my pain meant that he found some relief and gradually we were able to reclaim some of what was lost between us.

Peer support at its best provides the tribe that parents are in desperate need for, especially those parents struggling with their mental health. In the Digital Age we have lost the connections and communities that used to bond us together. No longer do villages raise children, instead many parents are now facing the daunting task of raising their children in ever-increasing isolation and their mental health is suffering as a result. The community of neighbours that was around when I was growing up is now a rare thing. Most people barely know their neighbours, never mind feel comfortable enough asking them to help in times of need. We are so secluded and closed off, afraid of what others might think of us that we are losing this crucial support network. Peer support never needed a label of its own before, it was an inherent part of life and it is disturbing to think that while peer support has never been needed more than it is now, it is fundamentally lacking in today's society.

If you are reading this now and are in need of a community who understands your struggle, I would urge you to find your local support group. PANDAS Foundation is a charity that works with families going through a perinatal mental illness. You can also find more information on how to get support in the Part Three of this book or check out the Resources section. Go find your tribe, find those who are where you are or who have been where you are and find a way through it together. You will find that you are not alone and that there is hope. The only way we can really defeat mental illness is through connection and togetherness. By opening up to others and sharing our experiences, we can break the isolation we have all become so entrenched in.

Don't get me wrong, running PANGS hasn't all been plain sailing. It comes with the territory that there will be tensions and difficulties when discussing some very personal experiences. But for the most part the group is a supportive and caring community. To have that company and shared experience made the long nights feel a little less lonely and the journey to recovery a little bit smoother. On occasion the group has been able to save lives and while I am immensely proud of that fact, I also don't think it is something we should need to do. There should be services and support for families to prevent it getting to that stage.

One of the biggest benefits of the group has been the sharing of knowledge and resources that many people may not have been able to find. As an example, I had no idea that the perinatal psychology department at my local hospital even existed and neither did my GP. It was only when someone who had accessed the service shared their story in the support group that I was able to go to my doctor and ask for a referral. As the group shared their stories of the therapies and techniques they had tried, a list of resources began to grow.

It was then that I realised that we needed a public facing service for anyone who might not feel comfortable sharing in a support group but who have the same need to access the resources the group often provided.

I created the PANGS website (www.wearepangs.com) which became a signposting and resource site that could direct parents to the services they needed, the self-help techniques they could use and information how to advocate for their loved ones. I put the NHS care pathways on the site so that parents could print them out and bring them to their GP to make them aware of what services were available and how they could be referred.

I also began to publicly blog my own experiences to help break the stigma surrounding mental health and to allow people to see how it affects the lives of not just the parents but the children, the extended families and the wider community. Through the blog I document my journey through mental illness including treatments I have tried and self-help techniques that have made a difference to me. I find that my blog attracts not just those suffering with perinatal mental illness, but people from across my community suffering with all kinds of mental illness. It is also used as a resource for health professionals to train their staff.

I became a kind of spokesperson for anyone who was suffering and in need of help, speaking at public events and staff training days at hospitals. I regularly get private messages asking for advice and support and while I do my best to help when I can, I'm conscious that I am not a health professional and that there should be professionals available to provide this service.

PANGS has become so much more to me than 'just' a support group, a blog or a website. It has become a calling and it has changed the whole course of my life. It was through the support group that I found out about the treatment options that were available out there. It also opened the door to campaigning for better services and brought a number of wonderful people into my life who are leading the charge for families in need of help. One of the campaigns we are working on is to bring a recognised peer support model to Northern Ireland which will train volunteers to run their own peer support groups. If we have a peer support group in every community, the effect would be enormous. No longer would those families who are suffering be stuck in their silence and isolation but would be free to join others and travel the path to recovery together. It would rebuild that lost network of support and connection and give parents a space to explore the difficulties they are experiencing in a safe and trusted group. PANGS NI is proof that peer support works and it is a service that every parent every where should have access to.

It saved my sanity and gave me a point to anchor myself to when the storm that is mental illness threatened to blow me away. I believe everyone needs that anchor and I'm determined to see it happen in my lifetime.

Chapter Eight - Rewind Therapy

In the months after starting PANGS, I began to ask the members what therapies they had tried and found helpful as anxiety was still playing a huge part in my life. I was determined to get on top of it once and for all and reached out for guidance on what to try next.

A group member told me of a midwife in another Trust who ran a Birth Afterthoughts clinic for women who were having mental health difficulties. Unfortunately because I hadn't birthed in that Trust I was unable to access the service. That didn't stop me though. Now that I had found my fight, I wasn't going to let anyone tell me what I couldn't have or couldn't access any more. My health and my daughter's health depended on it and so I pestered that poor midwife until she finally agreed to see me privately.

At my first session, I explained what had been going on, the endless days of anxiety, the constant replaying of my daughter's birth and I wept with grief as I explained that I couldn't imagine ever being pregnant again, knowing that I would not survive mental illness a second time. I had gone from wanting a football team of babies to not seeing how I could ever allow myself to become a parent again. I explained my guilt that I wasn't a better mother and my sadness that all of those special memories of her as a baby had been passing me by.

She took a breath, looked me in the eye and told me that I was suffering with birth trauma-induced PTSD (post traumatic stress disorder), my brain's very normal reaction to what it perceived to be a traumatic experience. PTSD used to be known as shell-shock and was first recognised in soldiers returning from World War I. The re-experiencing of the traumatic event through flashbacks, severe anxiety, outbursts of anger or sadness, are all normal symptoms of the brain's attempt to process the event and are beyond the sufferer's control.

She told me it wasn't my fault, that I wasn't a bad mother and that most of all, I could be helped. This wasn't a weakness or a flaw in my character. It was an illness, and like all illnesses I wasn't to blame. This wasn't something I had chosen or had failed to cope with. It was a disorder that needed treatment and now that I had a diagnosis, treatment could begin.

When I heard this, I cried so hard I thought I might be sick and then felt this weight lifted from me. We began a process called Rewind Therapy, a treatment which allows the brain to process traumatic memory and release trauma in the body (for more information see Part Three). It took just three sessions. I was so relieved that I finally found something that had worked but also so angry that this diagnosis and treatment hadn't been explored with me in the beginning with my GP. By the time I began Rewind therapy, my daughter was almost two years old. Those were years I was never getting back. Years that I spent living in a dark hole, a shell of who I once was. How many other women were out there suffering long and needlessly when they could be helped so quickly? It was infuriating to think that three sessions of therapy were enough to settle the more intense reactions I'd been having and allowed me to live a mostly calm and normal life. Gone were the flashbacks and the need to replay and talk about my birth experience. The daily anxiety became less intense and eventually I was having more days without anxiety than with it. I could enjoy my daughter and spent the last few months of my career break thoroughly immersing myself in motherhood and loving every minute (even the sleepless nights and tantrums!).

The treatment was so effective that six months later I was (intentionally) pregnant with my second child. Before therapy, the thought of getting pregnant again was so terrifying for me that you might as well have asked me to jump out of a plane with no parachute. And in a way that what it was like. I had no idea if my mental health would hold up and if I would be able to cope with two children while unwell. But the therapy was so successful that I felt strong enough and brave enough to face the uncertainty, knowing that if I became unwell again I had so many more resources than I had first time round. I had gone from a place of abject terror to a place of, not quite excitement, but enthusiasm all the same. I had spent two years mourning the children I thought I would never have and trying to make peace with Alexis being an only child. I felt guilty and weak to allow fear to prevent me giving Alexis a sibling. I didn't want to be that example for my daughter to follow, to let fear get in the way of the life you want. Rewind therapy got me back to a place of rationality and helped rebuild my confidence in my ability to cope. Five months later, my husband and I took the plunge.

Chapter Nine - Loss and Gain

Even though we had conceived our daughter quite quickly, I didn't expect to fall pregnant again straight away and yet two weeks after making our decision, here we were staring at two blue lines on a test. I felt this bubble of excitement mixed with panic well up in my chest. I paced the floor of our living room, half giggling, half hyperventilating and torn between happiness and fear.

What if became ill again?

I wonder what he or she will look like?

How can I cope with two children?

I can't wait to tell Alexis that she's going to be a sister.

What if I become ill again?

Never one to be able to keep a secret, we told our families straight away. They hated this, wondering why we didn't wait until our twelve week scan like everyone else to make sure we were out of the 'danger zone' of the first trimester. My logic had always been that if we were unfortunate enough to lose the baby, we would need the support of our families, and just like mental illness, miscarriage isn't something to be hidden away. It was another stigma designed to keep people isolated and alone during a difficult time because it was uncomfortable for society to acknowledge.

Unfortunately, three days after finding out we were pregnant I began to bleed and lost the baby shortly after. I can rationalise to myself that it was very early in the pregnancy and the baby would barely have had a shape. I can try to convince myself that it was just a bunch of cells at that stage and it was perhaps a blessing to have lost it so early on before it became something 'more'. I can do all those things but that will never make me forget that that baby was due to be born on 6th July 2015. It doesn't stop me wondering if it was a he or a she, or if it would have had it's sister's big brown eyes. We may not have lost a fully formed baby, but we lost the possibility of one and all the hopes and dreams that came with that. I became a mother the first time I saw those two blue lines and regardless of how and when the possibility of that baby ended, it did end and that was something to grieve. I was also overcome by the most horrendous guilt for having had reservations about being pregnant again. That pang of panic when the test was positive, that seemingly selfish concern for myself and my wellbeing. I began to think that perhaps I hadn't really wanted the baby at all and my body, recognising this, decided to end the pregnancy. I understand now that this was, of course, ridiculous and that there was nothing I did or didn't do to cause this loss.

Nothing prepared me for the trauma of that pregnancy ending in a physical sense. If I hadn't have taken a test I probably would have thought I was just having a heavy period and yet knowing that this familiar function of my body signalled the end of life was extremely difficult. I stood in my sister's bathroom with my hand on the handle of the toilet, knowing the pregnancy had ended and willed myself to flush. Even knowing that the baby was barely there, I couldn't bear the thought of it being swept into a sewer. It seemed so unnatural that this was the way I had to say goodbye. Even now years later, the first day of my period always takes me right back to that moment and each time I need to steel myself to flush the toilet even when I know there is nothing there. That's a difficult thing to relive month after month.

I found myself in the weeks after the miscarriage talking quite a lot about what might have been and suggested to my husband that we do something to commemorate the baby. I didn't want it to be forgotten about as if it didn't matter. As if it never existed. It might not have developed into a child, but I couldn't stop thinking about the child it would have been had we not lost it. I needed to do something for that child. The one who would never grow, say its first word, take its first step. The possibilities of its personality and hair colour and sense of humour. The idea of that child.

We went to our local garden centre and picked out an evergreen tree and two shrubs of heather, one pink and one blue. We planted them at the front of our house where we could see them every day. As I write this book I can see the evergreen tree right outside the window, grown from a tiny little shrub to around three feet tall, right about the height our baby would have been now. I take comfort from the fact that this tree is living in our garden and thriving. It gives the loss a semblance of meaning, that this tree is alive and growing in our baby's place. Not wanting to refer to the baby as 'the one we lost' or 'it', I decided to refer to him or her as Junior and the tree is known as Junior's tree.

Given my experiences with anxiety and depression, I knew that at this point I now had a choice. I could choose to dwell on what might have been or I could pick myself up and look towards the future and two months, almost to the day, of losing our baby, I found myself once again staring at two blue lines.

This time though, there was very little excitement. I was instantly consumed with gut-wrenching panic. Initially it was the very understandable fear of losing the baby, but as time went on and things were progressing as normal, it quickly became more than just normal nerves. I was once again right back into the throes of panic and anxiety, barely able to eat on some days and obsessed with my health. I would check my pulse regularly for palpitations, every twinge in my leg was blood clot, every dizzy spell was a stroke and I was utterly convinced that I was going to die in labour or shortly afterwards.

Worst of all, when I tried to imagine our baby earth side, I couldn't envisage a future with him in it. When I looked forward a few months in my mind, there was always a blind spot where he should be and it terrified me. I was convinced that my intuition was telling me he was going to die. That we both were. I would often tuck my daughter into bed then go and weep because she wouldn't understand why she didn't have a mother any more.

At its absolute worst, I would spend days in bed watching Harry Potter movies over and over again, because bed was the only place I felt safe and Harry Potter helped to give me courage. I know that sounds ridiculous but it was very comforting. I would imagine anxiety as a dementor and I just needed to learn how to produce a patronus charm to chase it away (if you have no idea what I'm talking about, seriously, read Harry Potter!).

I would get my husband to bring breakfast to me and my daughter before he went to work and we would cuddle in bed for the entire day watching cartoons, only leaving the bedroom to dash quickly downstairs for more food, panicking the entire way, before retreating back under the covers shaking. To say I felt tormented during those months was an understatement. I longed for him to arrive just for it to be over and yet, dreaded the day he would be born for the inevitable pain it would bring when one or both of us would die.

Halfway through my pregnancy, I began to seek help once again. This time I didn't visit my doctor, I was disillusioned with the help the NHS could offer me and I couldn't afford to be on a waiting list. I needed help now. I had spoken to my midwives and mentioned the anxiety but since there were no services to refer to me to, all I got were sympathetic smiles and reassurances that all would be well. I requested to be seen by the perinatal psychology team but despite repeated requests, the referral never came through. I finally decided the best course of action was to self-refer to a counselling service.

There was a local charitable counselling service near to where we lived so I went for an assessment, which basically consisted of me sobbing and spilling my guts out for an hour while a very kind lady listened and took notes. I began to see a counsellor every week after that and it was an enormous help. We did some somatic work which involved talking about my distress and then paying attention to how my body felt, where I was holding tension and how I was using my body to express myself. At the time it felt very strange but it helped to slow me down, to slow my racing thoughts and recognise how some of the physical symptoms I had been obsessing over for months had actually been caused by stress, not illness.

Knowing that I had someone impartial that I could talk to was a huge relief. I was very conscious that my husband was shouldering a lot of the responsibility for looking after me and our daughter at home, as well as trying to help me manage my mental illness, hold down a job and keep on top of everything else. There was only so much he could take. Having someone else I could vent to meant that the pressure lifted from him a little and as my mental health improved, life became a little bit easier. I should also mention that I would never have been able to go to counselling at all if it hadn't been for my family, in particular my big sister who gave up her time every week to watch my daughter. Without that support I never would have been to get that vital help.

One of the key benefits I found from regular counselling sessions was that I could set some of my worries aside throughout the week, scheduling them to talk to my counsellor about rather than dwelling on them constantly and getting trapped in these loops of negative thinking and worrying. Often, by the time my appointment came around I'd forgotten what the worry was, which proved to me that I could handle this stuff and cope. As my confidence in my coping abilities improved, I gradually began to realise that I could manage after all and didn't require the help of a counsellor any more. Once again, I began to prepare for the birth of my baby knowing that, even though I was still afraid, I could handle the outcome. I was still regularly posting in the PANGS support group and getting help from its members as well which helped massively. It was good to know that there were other women out there who weren't enjoying their pregnancies and were struggling, that I wasn't alone.

It is a difficult thing to admit, that you're not enjoying your pregnancy. There was a shame and a guilt when I thought about others who struggled to conceive and carry children to term and felt that I should be counting my blessings. However, I believe that everyone's problems are relative. Just because there are others worse off, doesn't diminish your own distress. In fact, the shame and guilt I felt for not being happier about my pregnancy just served to compound the problem and further limited my ability to recover.

In preparation for my son's delivery, I once again began practising hypnobirthing and found it massively lowered my stress levels and helped to ease the anxiety. The one thing it didn't help with was reliving my first birth experience. I would spend many nights wide awake from dusk to dawn thinking about what happened over and over again. This time, however, I wasn't having flashbacks to that day as I had been when I suffered with PTSD. Instead I was analysing every detail so that I could avoid the same experience happening again. I was so determined to have the birth I wanted, the birth I needed, so that I could have the best chance at good mental health after the baby was born. I would stay awake until the sun came up, covering every angle, preparing every response, anticipating every outcome. I spent so many evenings boring my poor husband to death with drills about what to do if I was offered drugs, what to do if I was getting stressed, if someone came at me with scissors for an episiotomy without asking my consent. He would climb into bed at the end of the day and I would give him pop quizzes.

"What do you do if I'm in the birthing pool and they ask me to get out?"

"What do you say if they ask you to leave and come back when labour is more established?"

He must have been tormented but it was the only way I could feel like I had any sort of control over what was about to happen.

I had found out through PANGS that the hospital I was birthing in ran a Birth Choices clinic for women who had had previous traumatic births. I asked my GP to be referred there for my antenatal care. My GP had no idea the clinic existed and wasn't sure what to do. I received an appointment for a regular antenatal clinic in the hospital I had birthed in before, the hospital that I couldn't drive past without a pang of anxiety. I called up and in no uncertain terms told them that I wouldn't be setting foot back in that hospital and that they needed to make the arrangements I had requested, to be seen at the Birth Choices Clinic in the hospital I had chosen to book in with.

Had I not been a part of PANGS, I would have no idea this clinic existed, nor would I have felt so emboldened to demand to be seen there, but I knew that my mental health and potentially, my life depended on it. It was one of the best decisions I made.

I was seen regularly by a consultant who supported positive birth experiences and believed in empowering women. Every time I went in with a concern, she put my mind at ease and knowing I had someone in my corner within the system was a big relief. She wrote on my notes that when I went into labour, I was to be assigned a Senior Midwife and having Birth Choices on my birth notes meant that whoever was assigned to me would know that I had a difficult experience previously.

Needless to say, as labour day approached I was getting more and more anxious. I began having regular contractions six weeks before my due date and unlike the Braxton Hicks I had had in my first pregnancy, these were strong, painful and regular but always stopped after a few hours, never leading to anything.

This meant that for weeks I was living with the pains of early labour which took me right back to my previous birth, not to mention the physical exhaustion of being in pain and still having to function for the sake of my daughter. I was beyond tired and the old fears began to seep in. Every time I bent over to breathe through yet another contraction, I recited my birth plan in my head, rehearsing all the things I would say and do, a plan for every possibility. I just couldn't relax. I felt like I was fighting for my life. If we didn't die in labour, I needed my mental health to hold up. I couldn't walk through that darkness again, not with two children to look after. I wouldn't survive.

Chapter Ten - Cooper's Birth

In comparison to the birth of my daughter, which seemed like a textbook delivery on paper and yet was profoundly traumatic, the birth of my son was the exact opposite.

I went into labour right on my due date after a day celebrating my nephew's christening. I climbed into bed at 10pm ready to sleep when I had my first twinge. I didn't pay it much attention given that I'd been having these pains for weeks on end. An hour later though we dropped Alexis off to her grandparents house and were on our way to hospital with contractions that were taking my breath away. We checked into labour ward at midnight, 8cm dilated and panic was coming thick and fast.

The moment we walked into the delivery suite, I handed a note to our midwife explaining our first experience and my struggle with anxiety. This wonderful woman sat down for a moment, read through everything then asked me how she could help me. It was so simple and yet I doubt she will ever understand the profound impact it had on me. I immediately trusted her to look after me and knew that she genuinely wanted me to feel safe and cared for.

At this point I was already frantic, pacing and crying, petrified that I would never leave this hospital. I told her that she needed to keep talking to me, to tell me everything that was happening, even if things were going wrong. I told her my imagination would think up the worst scenarios so I needed to know every detail to be able to cope. She really listened and that made such a difference.

As she filled the birthing pool for me, she left space for Eoin to care for me and he held me as we swayed together, trying to relax and allow our birth to happen unimpeded. She gave me gas and air which initially made me feel worse despite the calm it had provided me in my first birth. I kept repeating over and over again to Eoin:

"This is a double edged sword. It's helping with the pain but it's making me panic".

Gradually though, as I became accustomed to the floaty feeling I began to relax. I finally sank into the water and the warmth and buoyancy were like heaven to me. Just like my first birth, this relaxation in the water seemed to speed the process up and within minutes I was pushing at the midwife's instruction. I pushed for a short period of time when the midwife asked me if I would mind getting out of the water, she was concerned that the baby was in distress and wanted to have a look to see what was going on.

Unlike the first time round when I was manhandled out of the water with no explanation, this midwife openly explained why she was asking me to do it, and I understood that being in the water made it difficult for her to gauge what was going on. She was upfront and gave me a choice. At no point did I feel like I was being coerced and so, with difficulty, I climbed out of the pool of my own accord and climbed onto the bed to be examined.

At this point, as my son's head was crowning, things started going wrong. Even in my gas and air induced haze, I could hear on the doppler how slowly my son's heart was beating. I watched the midwife's face as her eyebrows knitted in concern and I heard her ask my husband to push the emergency switch. She explained to me that the baby was in distress and she just needed someone else in the room to assist. At that point I looked at husband. My unshakable, steadfast, rock of a man and watched the blood drain from his face as he looked down to where my son's head was beginning to emerge.

"What's wrong Eoin?"

"Nothing, everything's fine." He swallowed hard and gripped the bed rail.

"Please tell me what's wrong." I imagined the baby was dead or injured.

"Nothing, you just really need to listen to the midwife now."

She tells me I really need to get the baby out now.

"Nothing to worry about, he's just a bit stressed out so let's have a really big push."

I pushed with all my might and when I stopped, I looked back to Eoin who had turned a whiter shade of pale and had just begun to faint. The midwife caught him before he hit the ground. My immediate thought was (and I blame the gas and air for this!)

"I need to get up to Eoin, I need to make sure he's OK. My husband's on the floor!".

Seeing him so vulnerable and clearly concerned took away all my panic about myself and gave me the motivation I needed to get this baby out. No more fighting the contractions. No more letting fear hold me back. It was time to do this. I gave one almighty push and my son was born, a whopping 10lb 3oz and fit as a fiddle.

The second he was handed to me I had that rush of mother-love that I had missed out on first time round. I was instantly besotted and couldn't stop kissing his warm, wet head. The relief that it was over, the happiness that we had first of all survived and secondly, that we had that instant bond was such a departure from what I had experienced before.

As Eoin was helped onto a sofa by another midwife, I breathed a huge sigh of relief and felt stronger than I had in years. I had done it. We had done it. All the fear and apprehension leading up to the this day had been for nothing. Our baby was here, we were both safe and everything was great.

So you see, on paper his birth could have been construed as traumatic what with the emergency alarm going off, Eoin passing out, the baby's heart dipping dangerously low, and yet I found it so healing. There was only one difference between that experience of birth and my first. We had a midwife who was compassionate with her care and with her language. Not once did she make me feel like I was being dramatic, or like I was just a vessel through which my son was being born. She really took the time to care for me emotionally and physically. That was the difference. Something so small and easy to do and it made such a huge impact.

After our son, Cooper, was born she left us to enjoy him and to bond together, only interrupting to check if I needed any stitches. I did but this time hardly any. Once we had time to get to know our baby boy better, she sat beside me and asked me how I felt the experience went. I grinned from ear to ear and thanked her profusely for helping me get the experience I needed. She talked me through everything that had happened why certain decisions were made and I was so grateful for that. It meant I was able to spent the next few weeks enjoying my baby rather than questioning my birth.

I will be forever grateful to that midwife and everything she did for me. Anytime I am in the vicinity of the hospital I find myself hoping to bump into her so I can hug her and thank her again. She is what every midwife should be.

I left that hospital on cloud nine and things only got better. The anxiety I had suffered since my daughter was born three years previously had completely disappeared. I enjoyed my life for the first time in three years and I could see hope and happiness in my future. My bond with my children went from strength to strength and I finally felt like everything fit. Things were just perfect. Cooper was a dream baby who cried to go to bed at six o'clock and slept through until eight most mornings so I was having the best sleep of my life. I could leave the house, I could play with the kids, I could eat without fearing getting sick or choking.

The only cloud the sky of my life was the thought of the baby we lost. I would look at Cooper, so amazed and thankful to have him in my life and knowing that he was only here because we had lost the baby who would have been born two months earlier. I couldn't imagine a world without Cooper in it and I felt in turns sad and grateful that circumstances had played out the way they had. Our loss meant that this little boy could exist. It made me love him even more, if that as possible. He was my rainbow baby, the baby who healed the loss, who healed the anxiety and who made me whole again. Because of him I could finally be the mum I wanted to be and my relationship with my daughter flourished even more now that I was free of the seemingly unshakable anxiety.

Life was going great. But isn't there always a hitch?

Chapter Eleven - Accidental Baby

After my son was born, it was as if his birth had magically healed me. I went from being a constant nervous wreck to being able to enjoy life once more and I had no idea how that had happened. I have this vivid memory of taking a day trip with my husband and the kids to the seaside. The sun was shining, the sea air was invigorating and I felt this real sense of peace that I hadn't felt for many years. I smiled and tears welled up in my eyes as I realised that, for the first time since my daughter was born, I had woken up that morning and not thought about anxiety at all. I was at total peace and could see with such clarity how ill I had actually been. I cried as I realised that the illness had lost its grip on me and I was finally free. I felt like I could fly! I remember so clearly thinking to myself that, if I ever got lost in that darkness again, that this was the moment to remember. That this moment right now was the memory I would need to hold on to to see me through any tough times ahead. Little did I know, those tough times would reappear sooner than I had expected.

Following the birth of my son, my husband and I agreed that we would count our blessings and not have any more children. It felt right, just the four of us. If both kids were ill, they had one parent each to help. We didn't need a bigger car. We could book holidays which are always priced for two adults and two kids. I had always thought I would have a large family but I accepted that this was the right fit for us and things were so great, I didn't want to risk it all falling apart. I was grateful to finally put my experiences behind me and to be able to look forward with certainty that perinatal mental illness would never darken my doorway again. I never had to think about pregnancy or labour ever again, I could finally store away my birth experiences in the a box labelled 'The Past' and start looking to the future.

Through my own experiences and working with PANGS, I rediscovered my passion to help others. Every time a friend or family member became pregnant I was filled with this overwhelming desire to prepare them for birth and for life with a baby (without scaring the wits out of them in the process!). I really wanted to give others what I didn't have, a firm grasp on the options available to them. Cooper was ten months old when I decided to enrol on a degree through the National Childbirth Trust and University of Worcester to become an antenatal teacher.

During my first semester I was observing another antenatal teacher facilitate a group and I was so overcome by this longing to rewind and do my first birth over again with all this information at my fingertips. The course explored everything from pain relief options to coping strategies for life with a new born. It was done in such a way that their was no judgment of parents' preferences and everything was evidence-based which was a big draw for me. There were so many things I would have done differently first time around if I had been on this course and I was excited to be able to help others avoid the negative experiences I had been through.

Not long after this observation, I was sat in the middle of a breastfeeding exam (all theory, I wasn't expected to whip out the girls and demonstrate positions!) and I felt this wave of excitement. The kind of excitement you would get as a kid on Christmas Eve that starts as a ripple of butterflies in your stomach and wells up into your chest, almost catching your breath. I giggled to myself and thought "Weird, that only ever happens to me when I'm pregnant."

Stop.

Wait.

I couldn't be.

I began to furiously count up the days from my last cycle and realised my period wasn't due for another four days. I took a breath and told myself that I couldn't possibly be pregnant and I was being paranoid. I continued with the exam and went on about my day but I couldn't shake that feeling. That night after the kids were in bed, I told Eoin what had happened and he looked at me as if I had two heads. There was no way I was pregnant. I didn't need to take a test, it was all in my head. Yet I couldn't settle until I knew for sure so I drove to my local supermarket and bought a pregnancy test. I couldn't wait until I got home so I headed straight to the toilets and did the test. I walked to the car park with it up my sleeve, not daring to look until I was safely in my car and could check it in relative privacy. Sure enough, there they were...two pink lines, clear as day.

I began to freak out. Both my sisters were pregnant at the time and there were constant questions from family and friends if I was going to 'join the club'.

"No chance in hell!" I repeated regularly.

Yet here I was in the car park of Tesco, shaking, panicking, unable to comprehend how the hell this had happened. My first thought was to call my mum.

"Mummy," I sobbed, "I think I'm pregnant". I knew I was bloody pregnant. There was no doubt.

She talked me down as I tried to regain some sort of control over my breathing, assuring me that everything would be OK and that this baby was just meant to be. I don't remember how I managed to drive home in the state I was in but I remember opening the front door and my husband coming out to the hall.

"Well?" he said, knowing rightly I wouldn't be able to wait until I got home to take the test. I just burst into tears and said "I'm not ready for this."

He hugged me and despite not wanting any more children himself, he had a big, dopey grin on his face. He told me to think of the two we had and how amazing they were, to focus on the positives. It was a baby. It was the third child I always thought I would have. We would manage and everything would be fine. I wish I had been able to believe him but in that moment, and for a long time after everything felt the very opposite of fine. Again, we told our families straight away, only this time it wasn't in case we miscarried and needed support, it was in case I went into meltdown. With my previous two pregnancies I had time to prepare myself, to get my head on straight. This was such a shock and I just wasn't ready for it. Things had been going so well and I couldn't shake the thought that this was just asking for trouble. Surely this time around something would go wrong.

My sister-in-law, who had been trying for a baby had found out three days before that she was also expecting. Four babies in our family in the space of six months. I kept thinking the odds were against us, four women, four pregnancies, four babies. Surely something would have to go wrong with one of us, and I was convinced that someone was me. This wasn't helped by the fact that I was the last one to give birth so as I watched each baby delivered safely, I felt that statistics were not on my side. With every health baby born, it seemed to me that my baby stood less of a chance. I know how irrational that sounds but I found myself once again dreading labour, sure that one or both of us wouldn't make it.

I hated myself for not wanting to be pregnant, especially given how devastated I was when we lost Junior. I really wanted to relax and enjoy this pregnancy, to have hope that this was supposed to be, but I just couldn't. It was as though a switch had been flipped in my brain, taking all the happiness, joy and calm from my life and replacing it with gut wrenching panic and anxiety. Morning sickness triggered my health anxiety and once again I was spending every waking moment aware of every bodily sensation and wondering which one was going to kill me. I was so tired that I could barely lift my head and yet I still had to work, to look after my other two children, to get through the day when all I felt was dog-tired and absolutely hopeless.

I watched my sisters embracing their pregnancies and coping so well while I felt so incapable and fragile. I found some solace that my sister-in-law also didn't seem to be enjoying her pregnancy and it was a great source of comfort to be able to talk to someone who understood how I felt.

I hated myself for not being able to think my way out of this funk, especially as I had spent the last four years working on my mental health, learning all about how my brain worked and practising ways to manage my moods. None of this was helped when, at thirteen weeks pregnant, Cooper and I were involved in a car accident that sent me spiralling back down the rabbit hole of trauma and despair.

I was hit from behind by a Land Rover and careened into a car in front. I was immediately (and appropriately) consumed with panic as I jumped out of the car and ran round to the back seat to check my son was OK. I didn't realise until the next day that I had lost a shoe and had run over broken glass which got embedded in my feet. We were relatively unharmed, though I suffered pretty bad whiplash. However, shortly after the accident I began to lose my vision and the feeling on one side of my body. The doctors at the hospital couldn't figure out what was causing it and wanted to keep me in overnight. I had asked if I could have a scan to check if the baby was OK. I waited for hours before they agreed to let me walk over to the maternity unit to be checked over. I lay on the bed as the midwife moved the wand around my belly. There was a period of a few minutes when we could hear no sound nor see any movement despite the baby showing quite clearly on the screen. The sense of dread began to build and as I looked at the her little body unmoving, I realised then how much I wanted her and held my breath, waiting for signs of life. I stopped watching the screen and instead looked at the midwife's face as she frowned. I could see the thoughts move across her face, I could see her trying to find words to tell us the baby had died. She probed the wand deeper into my abdomen, circling and moving, searching for any sign of movement. Then there it was, the unmistakable sound of a heartbeat, racing along quite healthily, and as if to say "I'm here and I'm fine!" our little jelly bean baby jumped and wriggled non-stop for the next few minutes as the midwife checked everything else was OK. I saw the midwife breathe a sigh of relief and I shed a few silent tears, glad that all was well and promising to find a way through the anxiety for the sake of this little baby.

Back at A&E, the doctors decided that the unexplainable blindness and numbness was a stress response to the accident. I laughed at the irony. My brain which was so hyper-vigilant for any signs of illness, thought that the best way to help me cope with a traumatic experience was to make me think I was having a stroke. Well played brain!

After I was discharged, and very aware of my history of trauma, I spent the next few days resting and waiting for the panic and anxiety to set in. My plan was not to fight it, to accept it and let it run its course. I was very rational and aware of how my brain operated so I knew what to expect. It never happened. I remember telling my husband that the car accident might have been a blessing in disguise, the worst had happened and I had coped. I was fine, I wasn't traumatised, I had processed the event in a calm and logical manner and I had some confidence in myself and my ability to cope again. Best of all, it had put my pregnancy into perspective and I realised how important it was to get on top of my mental health once more so that I could prepare for the arrival of this baby.

Six weeks later though, as I was driving home from my mother-in-law's house, I was suddenly overcome by this overwhelming sensation that I was about to die. I was stopped at a traffic light with the kids in the car and I couldn't breathe. I had to keep shaking my hands and arms and didn't know why. I was desperate to get out of the car and scream for help. I didn't want to scare my children and I couldn't abandon them in the car so I called my husband and asked him to talk to me until I got home. Ten minutes later I was in the kitchen, clinging to Eoin and shaking so hard that my muscles ached, with my daughter asking me why I went "all jiggly" in the car. I quickly realised that this was just a very severe panic attack, the one I'd been waiting for since the car accident. I say 'just'. Anyone who has been through a severe panic attack will know that you may as well be dying because as far as your brain is concerned, that's what is happening. Your body is flooded with adrenaline and cortisol, all designed to keep you alive, to fight or flee, and when you've reached that point, the rational part of your brain switches off and you don't have access to logic.

This was the beginning of crippling panics attacks that on occasion meant that I couldn't get into my car to go to work, or I would be at work and would have to pull over several times on the way home because I thought I was going to pass out at the wheel. The worst attack I had saw me pull the car over at the side of a main road and get out to lie on the pavement, my 'logic' being that if I died there, someone would see me and be able to help my children who were in the back seat. So I began to avoid driving.

The problem with anxiety is that it makes you avoid the things you fear. The more you avoid them, the bigger the fear becomes until it becomes so big it starts to encroach on other parts of your life. At first I stopped driving distances longer than around five miles, the distance to my mum's house. Then I began avoiding motorways, then short trips to the closest shop until finally I only drove when I absolutely had to. I would make plans with my sisters or sister-in-law and cancel last minute, making some excuse. Sometimes I would be honest and say I was too anxious to drive and on several occasions they would come to me instead. But mostly, I would say one of the kids was sick, or I'd had a bad night's sleep and wasn't up to it. And so isolation began to creep in. It was when I began retreating to my bed again, watching Harry Potter on repeat, that I realised I needed help and once again sought out the wonderful lady who had treated my birth trauma before. Not only did I know that Rewind therapy would help with memories of the accident, but as my therapist was a midwife, I knew she could help me prepare my mental health for the birth of my baby.

I saw her every week for several months. We did work around the car accident, revisited my previous birth trauma and put together a mental health care plan so that I would be as prepared as possible for poor mental health should it continue after the baby was born.

I also chose to attend the Birth Choices clinic again. This meant I got to see my amazing consultant obstetrician, Dr Niamh McCabe, who put my mind at ease at every appointment, listening to my concerns and reassuring me that she would do everything in her power to ensure that we would have a calm and positive birth experience. Gradually I began to feel more in control.

In between my appointments at the Birth Choices clinic, I was seen by a community midwifery team at my GP surgery. On several occasions I mentioned the anxiety and asked to be referred to the perinatal psychologist. Most of the midwives I saw had no idea that this service existed or how to refer me on. Finally, fairly late in my pregnancy, I was seen by a wonderful community midwife called Hazel and a student midwife Suzanne. Expecting the usual lip service to my mental health, I had no expectations going into that appointment. I still planned to talk about how I had been feeling but assumed I would leave that appointment disappointed, like I had all the rest.

That appointment was the single most positive experience I had ever had with a community midwifery team. When I spoke about my difficulties, these wonderful women listened and made me feel that they really cared. Suzanne offered to be with me on my birthing day and Hazel set about referring me to psychology and for complementary therapies to help me feel more relaxed. I left that appointment feeling like I had finally made some progress, like someone cared for me and that things were going to be OK.

Two weeks later I was sat in front of the psychologist going over my history and explaining my concerns for the future. We both agreed that as I had been doing well with the therapy I was already in, that we would take a wait-and-see approach and review my mental health after the baby was born. I felt so reassured that if my mental health was suffering, I would be seen quickly. I now had a multi-disciplinary team of people from midwives, to my obstetrician and psychologist who were all aware of my situation and were poised, ready to intervene if needed.

I had done so much work and planning for my mental health that all there was left to do to have the baby and wait. You see, you can be as logical as you like and plan as much as possible but mental illness isn't a choice. It isn't something you can avoid by careful planning, you can only plan to mitigate the effects if it does show up. I think that is where a lot of the stigma surrounding mental health stems from. Many people think that it's an attitude problem, a choice to wallow or hide away. Many don't realise it is an illness like any other, and like any other illness it needs compassion and understanding.

Chapter Twelve - Luna's Birth

As the my due date came closer I found myself, not quite calm, but definitely more accepting of what was to come and generally more relaxed than I had been. I was ready for whatever was to come next and couldn't stand the anticipation. I just wanted to safely deliver my baby and finally be able to say that I would never, ever have to go through this again. Of course nothing is ever straightforward and I foolishly believed that as my first daughter was three days early, and my son was bang on his due date, that my final baby would be right on time. Boy was I wrong!

Ten days after my due date, on a Friday, I sat in front of a registrar I had never met before as my consultant obstetrician was on holiday. She told me I needed to be induced. She didn't ask me, she told me. Now don't get me wrong, she was a very pleasant woman who I'm sure had my best interests at heart, but being 'told' to do something strips away some of your power and makes you feel a bit more vulnerable. In the environment of a hospital, this is greatly amplified. After all, these people had spent years in medical school and practice. They were the experts and this was my baby's life we were talking about.

I tried to explain my anxiety around hospitals to her and how desperate I was to avoid being induced, especially since my husband wouldn't be able to stay with me outside visiting hours, even during the induction. It was enough to spark off a massive panic. Luckily for me I had spent the past year surrounding myself with knowledgeable and strong women who advocated women's choices based on the evidence provided, and I knew that going overdue only marginally increased the risk to me and my baby. I managed to push back on being induced that day and asked to wait until the following Monday. She said she 'couldn't let me go that long' but would agree to hold off until Sunday. Well thank you very much kind lady. You have been so gracious in 'allowing me' to have a semblance of control over my own body. Can you tell I was royally pissed off?

Not only was I told I would be induced on the Sunday, I wasn't actually given any information on what that involved. I was simply told that I would receive a phone call 'at some point after 6am' on the Sunday morning and be told to come in. First of all, I have two children at home who I needed to arrange childcare for...'some point after 6am' isn't good enough. Secondly, while I already knew from my degree course what induction involved, why was no-one taking the time to explain to me what would happen, why it would happen and what I could expect so that I could make an informed decision? Why was it assumed that I didn't have a decision to make, that I would just do as I was told? My consultant picked a really bad time to go on holiday!

I spent most of the next day either crying or on the verge of panic. I even contacted my consultant on Facebook and asked her advice. It wasn't until later that evening as I was weeping in bed that she responded to say that I could refuse to go and she would be back on Monday. If labour hadn't started by then we could talk through my options. I loved that this woman was in charge of my care. I'm so sad for all the women who aren't getting the same care. The sense of relief was amazing and I fell asleep comfortably, knowing that I had a reprieve if I needed it. I still had induction on my mind and was torn about whether to accept it. Even though I knew the risks to my baby were only marginally increased, I still worried that something might go wrong and that it would be my fault for not agreeing to the induction. I also felt some pressure from my family to just do it and get it over with. It is this kind of external pressure, however well-intentioned, that gradually chips away at a woman's confidence in her ability to birth and leads her to question her own judgment. Why are we doing this to women? Surely there has to be a better way?

Now before I continue, I want to point out that I have no issue with anyone who chooses to be induced. My decision not to do so was based solely on my fear of any kind of medical procedure. It just wasn't right for me and I wanted to do anything I could to avoid it. It saddens me that I have to make that disclaimer, that our society judges women so harshly on all of their choices that even when it comes to childbirth, we feel we need to apologise for our decisions. Fuck that. All I want is for every woman to have the benefits and risks laid out based on EVIDENCE and be allowed to make a decision based on fact. I want women to feel in control and empowered by their bodies and their birthing experiences, regardless of how that birthing experience plays out. There is no shame, regardless of how your baby came into this world. There is a hell of amount of shame on the professionals who underestimate your ability to understand your options and make an informed choice about your body and who disregard your choice in what happens to your body.

At 5am on the Sunday morning I woke up and lay for a while willing the baby to get her act together and start moving out! I knew that the hospital could call at any point to bring me in and I wasn't sure I had the strength to refuse induction.

I remembered from my course that there was some evidence that nipple stimulation could increase oxytocin levels and stimulate contractions so I thought, why not? Ten minutes later the Braxton Hicks kicked in. Ten minutes after that I realised that these weren't Braxton Hicks at all, this was the real deal.

I woke my husband and got the kids ready to go to my mum's house. When we arrived I forced my husband to eat breakfast, worried that if his blood sugar dropped that he would faint again in the delivery suite. I also wanted to delay getting to hospital for as long as possible. For a change, this wasn't because of my anxiety around hospitals, but because of my children. I had this overwhelming sensation once again that I was going to die in labour and I kept thinking that this would be the last time I saw them. I didn't want to leave them any sooner than I absolutely had to.

I eventually realised that if we didn't move soon, the baby would be born on my mum's living room floor and so I kissed the kids goodbye and walked towards the car, tears streaming down my face, hoping they would remember me. I understand now how totally irrational that was but, in the moment, it was all I could think of.

We arrived at the maternity ward and I paced through every contraction, unable to sit or be touched. Every time the pain built up, I felt the panic rise and that niggling thought 'You're going to die today' poking around in my brain. Each time I repeated to myself,

"Just breathe, all you have to do is breathe. Just keep breathing."

Eoin was a champion, quietly watching me, breaking the tension with a funny remark and reminding me to breathe every time I threatened to become overwhelmed. He reminded me of the hypnobirthing techniques and knew just when to hold me and when to leave me alone. He spoke to the midwives when I couldn't find the words and he timed my contractions. Every time I felt as though I was about to spin out of control I looked at his face. He was calm, relaxed and completely unafraid. Not only did this help me stay calm, but I realised that regardless of what happened, I could trust him completely to be the partner I needed in that moment and the parent our children needed if anything went wrong. I felt that I could let go of all the worry I was holding about what was to come next and trust him to take some of the weight for me.

We were moved to the delivery suite where I was finally able to have some gas and air and it was the sweetest relief. I got into a warm birthing pool and just rode those contractions with my mantra, 'Just breathe'. I had a fantastic midwife who stayed out of the way and let me get on with what I was doing, occasionally checking in to make sure everything was OK. I went into a world of my own and left Eoin to advocate for me if need be. As far as I was concerned, I wasn't in the room any more.

When it got to the pushing stage, I could feel my body squeeze and tighten and my first thought was to resist it as the anxiety began to resurface. I didn't want to push. I didn't want to have a baby. I didn't want to be here. But in a moment of clarity I realised that the longer I resisted, the longer this experience was going to last, and the more likely I was to run into complications. So when the next contraction came I went for it. After that push I realised that I couldn't hear what music was playing and the last song I remembered hearing was 'Only the Good Die Young' by Billy Joel. That line was repeating in my head and I frantically asked Eoin to tell me what song was playing now. I couldn't give birth singing 'only the good die young' in my head. It was a sign. An omen. I didn't have much choice though because the next contraction washed over me and again I just went for it.

At that point I had a horrible sensation that I can't quite describe while keeping my dignity intact. Needless to say it was about another bodily function! The sensation wouldn't leave me and I began to feel quite sick at the thought of it. I looked straight into Eoin's eyes, gripped both his hands and said in a frantic voice 'Oh God, I'm panicking'. This is it, I thought. This is when I die. I was so close and now this was the end, in a birthing pool on a Sunday morning. My husband, being the absolute champ that he is, leaned close and kept whispering in my ear 'All you have to do is breathe. Just breathe.' And with that came the next contraction.

I can't remember exactly how many pushes it took, I think around four before I felt that sweet relief as my baby girl was finally born. A midwife lifted her out of the water and before placing her onto my chest, unhooked the umbilical cord from around her neck. My first thought was how blue she looked and that she wasn't crying or moving. I talked to her, encouraging her to breathe.

"Come on baby girl, breathe for me. Come on, don't be scaring mummy."

I was very aware of the midwives' watching carefully and I vaguely remember one of them wiping her face. It must have only been around twenty or thirty seconds before she finally took a breath and began to whimper but it was the longest time of my life.

Everyone immediately sagged with relief and I lay back cuddling my little wet, warm bundle of wrinkles. She was the image of her brother and sister, with big brown eyes and sticky-out ears. Unlike Alexis where I had no feeling of love at all, or like Cooper were I was overcome with love, with Luna it was different. It wasn't an all-consuming love nor was it an absence. It just...was. It felt right to have her here, in much the same way that it felt right to have arms or legs. She was part of me and didn't need a gush of love or a fanfare to announce her arrival. I realised that although this was the first time I was holding her, her 'birth' as such had happened many months before, after the car accident when we waited with baited breath for her to show signs of life on the scan. Her arrival earth side was just a milestone.

I finally had the birth I had dreamed of, relatively calm, quick, and in water. I had panicked but with the help of my husband I got it under control and I bossed that shit. Here I was, glowing with pride in myself, love for my baby and gratitude for my husband. I felt like Superwoman. If she had been my first baby, I would have done it a hundred times.

Chapter Thirteen - Back into the Mire

For the first few weeks after Luna was born, I was very vigilant for signs of anxiety and depression. Eoin made sure I was eating well and sleeping as much as I could. He had a routine in the morning of taking the kids to school and daycare then returning to make me a smoothie packed with fruit, vegetables, a probiotic, iron and a vitamin pill. This was followed by a short nap while he looked after the baby then a breakfast of boiled egg and toast. This helped massively with my postnatal recovery and I found myself feeling stronger than ever.

Always conscious of becoming too reliant on him, I challenged myself to do things like make toast before they became obstacles too big to face and I was surprised at how well I felt. I tend to find the immediate postnatal period difficult. The bleeding and the pain reminded me of the miscarriage, but also of those dark winter nights I spent after Alexis was born, in a state of constant terror wondering if everything I was feeling was normal. I was so glad this time round that after two weeks I felt almost back to my old self.

Mentally I thought I was doing OK. I had my moments but I was managing and I knew I had the perinatal psychologist holding a space for me if I needed it. I genuinely didn't think I did.

It wasn't until three months later that I realised that actually something was wrong. I'd been having anxiety but I thought I was dealing with it. I had the odd panic attack but that was OK, they'd been so regular throughout the pregnancy that I didn't expect them to disappear overnight. I thought it was just residual stuff and that once I had fully recovered physically, and settled into our new normal as a family of five, that they would go away. I was wrong.

I made sure that I openly talked to Eoin and both of our families about how I was feeling. One night, I was explaining to Eoin that while I was feeling on edge most of the time, I didn't think I needed help.

"Michelle," he said, "you haven't left the house in four days. You're afraid to walk down the driveway to put something in the bin in case you die. You won't take the kids to the park across the street because you can't be outdoors alone. That's not normal."

Oh God, he was right. I had become afraid of leaving the house, but also afraid to be at home alone in case something happened to me. I was relying on Eoin working from home more and more, and shook with anxiety on the days he went into the office. I hated being alone, but found it so difficult to get out of the house to go be with people. How did I not realise how bad things had got? How did I miss this? Had anxiety just become so entrenched that this was just who I was now? I had been talking about what I had been feeling. I had been so aware of where I was with my mental health. Why did I not ask for help sooner? I spoke to my mum, my sisters and my sister-in-law and told them how I had been feeling and they all agreed that calling the psychologist was probably a good idea. Even then I still felt reluctant but with a nudge of encouragement I made an appointment.

It was a sign of how bad I was that when I arrived for my appointment I spent my time in the waiting room feeling like I was having a heart attack and debating running over to A&E for help. I managed to hold it together and when Andrew, the psychologist came to meet me in reception I was beginning to calm down.

When I sat down in his office, a whole well of anxiety just erupted out of me, things I didn't even realise I was feeling. I told him about an occasion where my son was ill and needed to go to A&E and how I tried to make my husband take him because I couldn't face the drive. My baby boy had needed me and I felt like a total failure. I did take him myself in the end but had a horrific panic attack on the motorway and felt like I was going to lose control of the car and kill us both. I explained how being outside made me feel disorientated and how I had a sensation that I was shrinking when I was outside alone. I told him how I refused to lock the bathroom door in case I collapsed and a paramedic needed to get in. I hanged my shame as I told him how I explained to my five year daughter the process for calling 999 in case of an emergency, trying to covertly teach her how to get help if I had a heart attack or a stroke. I had always been so conscious not to pass my shit onto her and here I was prepping her for some imaginary catastrophe that might befall me. How had I not realised how bad I was?

I was expecting him to talk me through a plan of action, to arrange an appointment to begin therapy with him but he told me that unless I was an in-patient I couldn't access his service.

What?

Why was this only being explained to me now? He suggested referring me on to the Adult Mental Health team at my local hospital but wasn't sure how long this would take and he offered to see me in the meantime to bridge the gap.

Four weeks later I was sat in another office, in another hospital explaining to a mental health social worker how agoraphobic I had become and how I was walking around in a state of constant anxiety most days. After an hour and half of gut-wrenching exposure and vulnerability, she looked me square in the eye and said:

"Mrs Bradley, I can see that you're going through a really rough time. You seem really aware of what's going on with your mental health and you are really good at identifying what you need to recover. If you hadn't just had a baby, and if you hadn't had suicidal thoughts in the past, I don't think you need to access this service."

Come again?

"I'll refer you on to the Psychology team anyway."

This really pissed me off. First of all, I am quite fortunate to have the ability to talk about my mental health quite candidly. Explaining that you wanted to shoot yourself in the head isn't an easy thing to say to a total stranger, particularly a social worker and all the fear that brings up about having my children removed from my care. How many people had this woman seen who didn't disclose their darkest thoughts and were shooed out of her office with a pat on the back and a "You'll be grand"?

Secondly, how bad do I need to be to get help? Isn't fearing death twenty four seven bad enough? Isn't being unable to leave my house bad enough? Aren't the intrusive thoughts of stabbing myself with a knife while making dinner bad enough? What exactly was "bad enough" to be taken seriously? It is a real bug bear of mine with the health service that the minute you show any sign of having educated yourself about your condition you're either labelled a self-diagnosing Google doctor, or you're assumed to be smart enough or competent enough to fix yourself. I was infuriated, not just for myself but for all the people, men and women, postnatal or otherwise who were desperately reaching out for help and this was what they were getting. It is no wonder that suicide is the number one cause of death in women in the first year of giving birth. Can't they see the impact they are having? Not just on the parents but the lifelong impacts on the children of parents with mental health difficulties? Why aren't they doing better!?

A few weeks later I, being one of the lucky ones to slip through the guarded gates of mental health services, sat in an office for my third mental health assessment in two months. This process is absolutely exhausting, having to rehash your entire history to yet another stranger in the hope that this one would get it, that this one would be the one to help. You need to have energy and strength and determination to navigate this system, three things that anyone with a mental illness will tell you is in short supply. This is the point when people give up. This is the point where they think there really is no hope. To have to go through these gruelling assessments and then to go home with your trauma and distress and have no follow-up or support to help you find equilibrium again is heartless and cruel. This is when you are at your lowest. This is the point I had been at before but this time I had an advantage and it was an advantage that I fully credit with preventing me spiralling down into the black pit once more.

What was my advantage? That memory of being at the seaside with my family when the cloud finally lifted and I felt peace. That moment when I realised this feeling of hope and happiness was as real and as valid as every negative emotion I had felt in the years previous. I had the wherewithal during that moment to focus on it, to store it somewhere in my memory that I could access it easily if I needed to. That moment saved me. I had hope because I had been through it before and I came out the other side. That is the hope that I want to share with everyone out there who is feeling lost. If you are reading this right now and feeling in your heart of hearts that there is nothing good or positive in your future to look forward to, just hang on. Fight for yourself. Find the help you need even if you have to see a hundred professionals to get it. You are worth it. You will get better. You can beat this. I know because I have.

That memory of that day by the seaside strengthened my resolve and on I forged with this third assessment and was initially offered twelve sessions of CBT therapy, to be reviewed at the end to see if it had helped. I was relieved to have a plan in place and took comfort that the next few months would undoubtedly help me to feel better and that I would start to enjoy my life again. And still I thought of others like me who had been turned away from this service and anger bubbled inside me at this lottery of care. I had once again been 'lucky' enough or at least, determined enough to get help. My heart broke for all those who had exposed themselves during the most vulnerable time in their lives in order to get help, and who had had the door slammed in their faces.

I began CBT therapy in January 2018 and gradually began to regain control over my thoughts, my emotions and most importantly my panic. I learned to intervene when the cycle of panic spun me out of control and over time the frequency and severity of the panic attacks decreased greatly. Therapy had raised some unresolved issues from my past including the sexual abuse and although the panic disorder was coming under control, I was finding myself more and more triggered about events in my past. I also found myself suffering from depersonalisation, a lack of feeling or connection to my emotions and to those around me. Although the panic had massively reduced, I felt like my life was happening to someone else, like I wasn't a part of it. I would watch myself playing with my children, watch myself enjoying them but I couldn't feel it. It was like watching my life on a TV screen, like it was happening to someone else. My therapist and I agreed that rather than end our sessions and leave these issues unexplored, that she would transfer me to another therapist who would be best placed to help me explore these issues.

I began therapy with this psychologist and after a few months of exploring these issues I can safely say that while I am not now, and probably will not ever be fully free of anxiety and mental illness, it is at a very low level. I have occasional bad days but they are much fewer and farther between and no longer completely overwhelm me. I have confidence in myself that I can navigate the difficult periods and if I feel myself begin to slip, I have a range of tools and a network of support to help me through. I have come such a long way from that trembling, seemingly incapable woman who had just given birth six years ago. While mental illness has been hell to go through, I feel stronger and more resilient than ever before. More importantly, I am also now that expert so that if my children are ever unfortunate enough to suffer, I can guide them through it. That is something of great value. Every cloud has a silver lining.

It has been a long six years since I was first diagnosed and such a lot has happened. I have gone from the absolute depths of despair to the giddying heights of joy and everything in between. I have had to work hard to find the help I needed and work even harder implementing the different tools I have learned but most of all, I have learned so much about my own capabilities and my ability to cope. If someone had told me back in those early dark days when the act of making toast seemed insurmountable that I would not only be happy once more but that I would have achieved so much because of the difficulties I faced I would not have believed them. Since my struggles began I have set up a thriving support network for others going through similar experiences, I am part of a volunteer group who are actively trying to improve perinatal mental health services in Northern Ireland. I have started my own business, written a book and have seen many of my lifelong goals achieved. I have gone from feeling completely incapable and broken, to feeling resilient, strong and proud. I don't say any of this to boast. I say it to you, the person reading this book who may be feeling how I felt, who may not be able to comprehend the strength you have, who may not be able to see a way out of the darkness. I have been you and I am living proof that there is always hope. Keep fighting for it.

Chapter Fourteen - Breaking the Stigma

Over the past six years as I've struggled with my mental health, it has become more and more apparent to me that many people just don't understand mental illness and the impact it has on individuals, families and communities. The stigma around mental health pervades our society to its core, especially when it comes to birth and parenting. Every day we are judged for our decisions and actions and pitted against one another in the so-called 'mummy wars'. If we had drugs in labour we're weak, c-sections are the quitters way out, women who birth without pain relief are hippies or martyrs. Do you breastfeed? Bottle-feed? Combi-feed? Regardless of how you choose to feed your child you will be subjected to some form of shame. The same goes for sleeping, parenting style, disciplinary practices. We can't do right for doing wrong. It seems that from the moment you test positive on a pregnancy test, everyone and their mother wants to tell you what you need to be doing, or point out what you are doing wrong.

It begins before you even have your baby. Is your BMI outside of normal range? You're putting your baby at risk. Don't get stressed, it's bad for the baby. Don't eat that, it's bad for the baby. Sleeping on your back? Bad for the baby. And it doesn't stop once the baby is born. Are they a 'good baby', meaning are they sleeping? Don't hold them, they'll never want to be put down. Don't answer as soon as they cry, you'll spoil them. Get them off the breast and onto a bottle so they aren't reliant on you. Not only are we expected to be perfect parents with all our shit together but we're judged on whether our babies are doing what they are 'supposed' to be doing i.e. sleeping and eating bang on schedule and generally behaving like perfect little angels. Does anyone actually have one of these babies? The pressure is immense.

It doesn't help that there is so much conflicting information that it would make your head spin. Everyone is frightened of doing it wrong and fucking up their kids. Many don't even consciously question why they use one parenting style over another or whether it's even right for them and their family. We want the world to see that we are confident parents who are doing everything 'right'.

We have created this society where we expect so much and support so little. Gone are the days of several generations of women looking after each other, supporting each other and helping each other to raise their babies. We now parent in isolation, behind closed doors only showing the happy, 'perfect' moments of our lives through our social media accounts. We create this postcard view of our lives online, for the world to see how great everything is and how fine we really are.

So what happens when we aren't fine? There is no longer any space for parents to admit they are struggling. Even when parents do own up to feeling less than fine, the support networks are not in place to assist and so they are left to figure things out on their own. When I was struggling after my first child was born, I initially didn't want to tell anyone outside of my family circle because I was worried that they would think I was a terrible mother. I felt like a terrible mother and I was trying to find a way to be better. I couldn't bear the thought of the outside world confirming what I thought I knew.

There are several layers to this. First of all I was having intrusive thoughts that I found difficult to put into words. I would often walk down the stairs and an image would flash into my head of me dropping the baby and her head cracking on the floor. Or I would be making dinner and imagine stabbing myself with the knife. Now here's the thing...intrusive thoughts aren't intentional thoughts. I had no intention of dropping my baby or stabbing myself. These thoughts would come unbidden to the forefront of my brain and haunt me through the day. I didn't know how I could explain that to a doctor without worrying that they would call social services and have my baby taken away.

I also knew that I would jump in front of a bus to save her life but I often looked at her and felt something was missing. I didn't get that butterfly feeling of love. I knew I loved her but I couldn't feel it. I often told my husband that I didn't think I loved her enough and that she would be better off with someone who did. I went to playgroups and toddler mornings, and watched other people with their kids and wondered what was wrong with me that I wasn't enjoying motherhood. Any time we had a visitor who would lift the baby and coo over her, I would wonder if they loved her more than I did. Why wasn't I feeling anything except fear and anxiety? I know now that fear and anxiety were using all my mental resources, prioritising survival over emotion and effectively switching off my ability to connect with those around me. But at the time, I just felt I wasn't good enough.

I was also surrounded by people who seemed to have their shit together and were totally in control of their lives. I come from a family of strong women who are at the centre of their own family circles and I felt I wasn't living up to expectations. How was I to be a leader, a care-taker and a protector of my children when I couldn't even leave the house? Add to this the massive amount of guilt that my mental illness was increasing the risks for my children to have difficulties with their own mental and physical health.

The other reason I think many new parents don't admit how they are feeling is because we're all supposed to be feeling so grateful right? I mean, there are people in the world who can't have babies and would kill for what I had. And they're right in a way, I should be grateful, but that assumes I had a choice in the matter. My mental illness isn't something I chose. It isn't something I could just will out of existence or think away. That's the mistake most people make. That mental illness is just a bad attitude. If you feel like you can't get out of bed, you're lazy. If you can't face seeing people, you're flaky and unreliable. If you don't love your kids with every ounce of your being, you're selfish or heartless. I can't think of another single medical condition where we blame the sufferer for their illness. If you have cancer, it's not your fault, it's something that happens to you and you're given sympathy, support and comfort. If you have asthma, you are given an inhaler and a care plan. No one says, well have you just tried breathing better?

The catch-22 here is that all this judgment and lack of understanding prevents us from accessing the one thing we need in order to recover... connection. Disconnection, isolation and lack of support are all the things that feed mental illness and keep us stuck in its trap. The only way we can come through it is to reach out to others, to share our experiences, to be able to admit how we are truly feeling however uncomfortable it is, and to be allowed to truly be ourselves as we are in the moment. By doing this, we can begin to tear down the walls that mental illness builds up and face it head on, knowing we have a support system in place to back us up and hold us when we are vulnerable.

By standing up and saying 'this is me and I need help' you are also giving others permission to do the same. Since I began my blog on PANGS NI, I have had so many people reach out to me to say they have felt the same way as I do and they are grateful that I opened up and shared my experiences. I made a very difficult decision when I started the blog to be as candid as I could be with my condition and censor none of the darker detail. It is only by shining a light on it that we can truly defeat it. In the beginning I worried that by opening up to the truth of how I was feeling, that I would also be opening myself up for criticism. We all know the trolls that lurk in the darker corners of the internet, ready to pounce on anyone who veers slightly away from the 'norm'. I made a promise to myself to accept the potential negativity I would encounter and bear it for the sake of the greater good. To this date, I have yet to encounter a single negative comment. Either the trolls agree with me or they just haven't found me yet!

I know there are many people out there who don't have the support, or feel safe enough to be candid with their feelings. There are so many people in desperate need of connection and this isn't happening because our society is uncomfortable with mental illness and we have lost all those innate skills we used to have to just be there for each other. We have become so entrenched in our isolation that many of us don't even know our own neighbours. How can we expect our new parents to reach out when they are effectively reaching out to strangers, strangers who can be so unforgiving and judgmental? And when you are given the most important job in the world, to protect and raise a healthy, well-rounded human being, the future of our race, how can we admit that we aren't coping? That is why I choose to document my experience. For all those who are unable to and yet still need to have a voice.

The problem we have in Northern Ireland, and it's reflected all across Western society, is that even in our health and social care systems we don't have the services for parents. I know so many midwives, obstetricians, GPs, and volunteers who are desperate to help parents on the ground and they have nowhere to refer them to. They can do very little without the infrastructure to back them up, and this is just not good enough, not just for the parents but for their children as well.

There is a growing recognition of Adverse Childhood Experiences (ACEs). The impact that the mental health of the primary care-giver has on a child reaches far into their adulthood raising their risk for mental illness, obesity, diabetes, heart disease and a range of other negative outcomes. The health of the baby begins with the health of parent. We could save our health service billions of pounds in future medical expenses by diagnosing and treating perinatal mental health early and treating it fully, and it doesn't take much. Throwing antidepressants at parents and sending them on their way is not good enough. Studies show that antidepressants are more effective if given in conjunction with talking therapies and other social prescriptions such as exercise in nature, pleasurable activity and connection.

Mental illness is a complex issue that drugs alone cannot cure. By the way, this is not a denigration of medicine. I think mental health medication has its place but it is not a cure-all for everyone. We need to address the core issues and take a whole-person approach to treatment and recovery.

By working together with the health service and the wider community to better understand mental illness, we can ensure that every parent gets the understanding, respect and treatment they deserve and set them on the path to recovery much quicker. It is my hope that by sharing my story, I can in some small way help to break the stigma and give a platform to all those who are suffering in silence.

Chapter Fifteen - Changes

In January 2018, myself along with four other volunteers came together with an idea. It was a simple idea and one that had been brewing in the back of my mind for several years. For many years in Northern Ireland, campaigns for better mental health services for parents seemed to be falling on deaf ears. Progress was slow and it was difficult to get the right people in the right rooms to move the issue forward. However, over the past year momentum has slowly been building and the time felt right to take positive action.

I had regularly wondered what might happen if we managed to get all the key stakeholders in the same room to explore the issue in depth, So when a message came through in early January in a group chat asking if anyone had any plans for Maternal Mental Health Week I tentatively pitched the idea of a Maternal Mental Health Conference. With only four months to prepare it seemed like an impossible task but the group was full of fierce, motivated and highly focused individuals so we decided to forge ahead. Why wait?

Over the next four months we put our heads together and gradually the conference began to come together and on 3rd May 2018, we opened to a sold out audience of nearly three hundred people made up of health professionals, parents and volunteers. To say the atmosphere in the room was palpable would be an understatement. By the end of the day everyone was incredibly psyched up and ready to go out into their own individual areas and make change happen. Never before had we seen something like this, where everyone came out of their respective silos and pledged to collaborate for a better future for our parents and children.

The conference was such a huge success that it has now become an annual event and has opened the doors for the campaign to build real momentum. The group were invited to talk with the All Party Working Group for Mental Health in Stormont, the seat of our government. The campaign work became much more powerful knowing that all the key players on the ground had banded together behind us to push for more, for better.

Our group is small, just five women but we are headstrong and determined to use this momentum to finally achieve what many others have been fighting for for years. We have three key asks:

1. A mother and baby unit so that no mother has to be separated from her baby if she needs in-patient psychiatric treatment

2. Specialist perinatal services in every health and social care trust across the country

3. The implementation of a peer support model so that volunteers can be trained to facilitate peer support groups that parents can access

These are services that are lacking, not just in Northern Ireland, but in many places across the world. Unfortunately, we just don't seem to place value on the mental health of parents and it is time that changed.

The charge has been led by Lindsay Robinson, a campaigner and blogger (Have You Seen That Girl?) who has used her own lived experience to highlight the desperate situation parents are in.

Seána Talbot, the President of National Childbirth Trust (NCT) has also spent the last twenty years fighting tooth and nail for better services and whose dogged determination is a wonder to behold.

Nuala Murphy, founder of Moment Health, has developed an app that allows parents to track their moods, check their symptoms and find support in their communities. She has been on the road constantly, fighting to make perinatal mental health mainstream. She has been a driving force for our group and a constant source of inspiration.

Catherine McCusker has been a long-term volunteer for NCT in Northern Ireland and is passionate about ensuring parents have the best start to family life.

Our little group is testament to the power of purpose and what can be achieved when like-minded people band together around something they are passionate about. By focusing on our common purpose we have been able to build on the work of those who came before us and bring maternal mental health into the spotlight. It is our hope that in the near future we will see our key asks become reality and thus improve the lives of countless parents.

During the planning stages of the NI Maternal Mental Health Conference I was on maternity leave with my youngest. I was in the middle of CBT therapy for agoraphobia, panic disorder and fear of driving. Having something to focus on became a real life line for me. Where before I felt I was drifting through my days in a haze of anxiety and isolation, now I had a purpose, somewhere to direct my energies, and my mood began to lift. Needing to attend meetings meant that I was forced out of the house and had to face my fears head on. The group were aware of my struggles and supported me throughout.

To say that the conference changed my life would be a fair assessment. It was while I was organising the various operational aspects that I rediscovered my love for event management. I was fed up in my part-time finance job and dreaded my maternity leave ending when I would need to leave my baby and return to the monotonous task of processing invoices. Organising the conference gave me the confidence I needed to strike out on my own and so I started my own event management company, ALC Events.

I thought long and hard about the types of events I wanted to organise and I wanted my focus to be on events that matter, that made a difference to the community. The first event I embarked on was the NI Positive Birth Conference. Going back to my birth trauma and the impact it had had for years to come, I wanted to help educate and empower parents to have positive birth experiences. I drew inspiration from the Maternal Mental Health Conference, focusing on bringing together health professionals, volunteers, private sector and parents to collaborate together and create a supportive community of people dedicated to positive birth.

This shift in my life from feeling adrift and purposeless to finding work that held meaning for me was a massive change. It meant I could work from home and be flexible around my family. I could pick and choose the work I wanted to do and I thoroughly enjoy taking an idea and bringing it to life. This change has made me a much happier and much calmer person which has had a ripple effect in my home. My children get to watch their mother being fulfilled and still be at home when they get in from school. My husband gets to come home to a wife who hasn't spent all day wallowing in her own anxious misery and desperate for solace.

My hope is that my company will be profitable enough in the near future to be able to come out of paid employment entirely and build something that not only supports my family financially but that continues to have a positive impact on my mental health and the wider community through the events I put together.

At the time of writing this book, my mental health has been on a steady path upwards. There have been moments of panic and despondency but they are much less often and I'm almost ready to finally put my demons to bed. I continue to share my experiences through my blog, through public speaking and campaigning and while I know that I am still on the road to recovery since my last baby was born, I have hope that in the near future I will be able to say I am healed. I hang on to that memory of the seaside and look forward to the day when I feel once again at peace. If you are reading this and you are in the throes of mental illness, I implore you to hang on to hope. In Part Three of this book I will share with you the techniques, therapies and services that you can explore to help you with your recovery, or to support a loved one through theirs. If these services aren't available where you are, keep looking for the services that are there. Reach out, speak to people, make a noise. Fight, fight and fight some more, even when you feel you have no fight left. A better life is within your grasp and there are more people than you know fighting right alongside you. Don't give up hope.

PART TWO:

PERINATAL MENTAL ILLNESS

This section of the book will describe the mental illnesses that are common in pregnancy and after childbirth. This is not intended to be an exhaustive list nor will it go into great detail but will give you an idea of the most common perinatal mental illnesses and how to spot them.

For further information on each of these conditions and more, check out the Resources section at the back of the book.

Chapter Sixteen - Antenatal and Postnatal Depression

It is estimated in the UK that 1 in 10 women will be diagnosed with a mental illness in pregnancy or in the first year after birth. Recent research by the NCT's Hidden Half campaign found that 50% of the women they surveyed reported that they had experienced mental health or emotional difficulties at some time during pregnancy or in the year after birth. That's 1 in 2 women.

Many of us will have heard of postnatal depression and it is often used as an umbrella term for all mental illness in expectant and new mothers but this isn't good enough. Personally, I didn't ask for help with postnatal anxiety because I had only been asked about postnatal depression and therefore didn't think my illness counted. In the beginning of my illness, I wasn't depressed, I was petrified. The labels we put on mental illness matter.

Antenatal depression in particular is not widely discussed or acknowledged. Many of the worries that expectant parents face are often discounted as pre-baby nerves or 'normal' anxieties. It is also often put down to fluctuating hormones, and while hormones do play a part in our moods, it doesn't account for everything related to depression.

Postnatal depression is more well known and documented though the symptoms are much the same.

How can you tell if you are suffering with antenatal or postnatal depression?

Sufferers will often describe perinatal depression as, rather than being a time of joy and excitement, pregnancy and the postnatal period become a time despair, hopelessness and anxiety.

Symptoms of Antenatal or Postnatal Depression

- Crying for no apparent reason
- Feelings of guilt or worthlessness
- Hopeless about the future
- Lack of energy, finding it difficult to get of bed and face the day
- Relationship worries (e.g. worrying their partner may leave before or shortly after the baby is born)
- Becoming withdrawn or hostile to those closest to you
- Feelings of hostility or indifference towards your pregnancy/baby
- Conflict with parents: pregnancy can often stir up emotions about their own upbringing
- Isolation
- Feelings of despair or distress outside the normal 'lows'
- Difficulty sleeping
- Fear of seeking help
- Irritable and angry
- Reduced appetite or increased appetite (comfort eating)
- Loss of concentration
- Intrusive thoughts, thoughts about death or thoughts of suicide

There are different theories on what causes antenatal and postnatal depression. It is most likely a combination of several of the below.

Physical

- Hormonal changes: pregnancy, childbirth and breastfeeding are times of great hormonal change in a woman as the body grows, nourishes and births a baby. This can cause changes in mood as well as physical changes in the body that may be uncomfortable or unsettling.

- Nausea: in pregnancy, nausea can cause a lot of mental distress, especially if it persists for the length of the pregnancy or is severe (a condition known as hyperemesis gravidarum)

- Iron and zinc deficiencies: these have been linked to depression in pregnancy as the body may become deficient. Eating plenty of iron and zinc rich foods is very important as well as Vitamin C to help the body absorb the iron.

- Changes in appearance: pregnancy and motherhood take a natural toll on how our bodies look. We may gain weight, lose weight, lose hair after pregnancy and our skin can change. All of this can make us lose some of our confidence. Especially in today's society were a great emphasis is placed on a woman's appearance, the process of becoming a mother and finding yourself with a body that feels different from usual can be very upsetting.

- Sleep: discomfort during pregnancy, and the normal frequent night wakings of a baby mean that sleep is often interrupted or you wake feeling unrested. Sleep is a crucial process that allows our bodies to heal and our brains to process the events of the day. When this is disturbed, the effect can be extremely detrimental

Emotional

Becoming a parent is one of the biggest transitions a person can go through in their lifetime. Every pregnancy, birth and baby are different and each comes with its own set of challenges whether this is your first baby or your tenth. Problems within relationships may be magnified, you may have other children at home who will need to adapt to a new sibling or you may be concerned about your job or financial situation. All of these stresses can be contributing factors in depression. If you have suffered a miscarriage or still birth, this can bring up feelings of grief and sadness as well as fear for the current pregnancy.

While in most cases antenatal depression will resolve before the birth of the baby, it is estimated that up to a third will continue and evolve into postnatal depression. It is important to recognise both conditions early in order for speedy diagnosis and treatment. It is important to note that perinatal depression is 100% treatable and in most cases can be resolved quickly with early intervention.

Chapter Seventeen - Antenatal and Postnatal Anxiety Disorder

Antenatal and Postnatal Anxiety Disorder

While anxiety is often lumped into the symptoms of depression, anxiety disorders can and do exist on their own without depressive symptoms. It is often only when anxiety reaches a point of crisis that depressive symptoms appear.

When we talk about anxiety, we are not talking about the normal every day worries and concerns. While anxiety plays a role in our daily lives (preventing us from stepping out in front or buses or running with scissors), the fight-or-flight response can become hyper-vigilant, always on the alert for danger. When this happens, seemingly innocuous events can trigger anxiety or panic attacks as the brain perceives threats all around.

How does anxiety work?

When faced with danger such as an aggressive dog, our brain prepares our bodies to react in one of four ways.

- Flight: run away from the danger

- Fight: fend off the attack

- Freeze: stay still in hope that the danger will pass by

- Flop: faint, giving the impression of death so that the animal will leave us alone. This is also triggered if the brain suspects that you cannot survive the attack, thereby preparing for a painless death through unconsciousness.

The brain assesses the situation and reacts in a fraction of a second, flooding your body with stress hormones (cortisol and adrenaline), sending blood coursing to your major muscles groups to prepare to fight or run away, dilating your pupils, amongst many other symptoms. This is the feeling of panic. The problem with an anxiety disorder is that the brain can't tell the difference between a real threat and a perceived threat. With anxiety disorders, the smallest thing can trigger a panic. For me it was my health. Any change in my body, any new sensation however small, would trigger a panic attack. For others it could be a smell that reminds them of a time they felt unsafe or intrusive thoughts of danger.

Emotional symptoms of anxiety

- Feeling anxious, nervous, or afraid most of the time

- Feeling like something awful is about to happen

- Feeling tense, uptight, unable to relax and on edge

- Feeling woozy, detached, unreal or strange

- Feelings of panic or terror

- Constant obsessive worrying

- Racing thoughts

- Dwelling on worst case scenarios/catastrophising

- Finding it difficult to carry out simple tasks

- Pacing, unable to sit still

- Talking more quickly than usual

- Snappy, irritable or angry behaviour

- Drinking or smoking more regularly

- Negative self-talk (I'm losing control, I'm making an idiot out of myself, I'm having a heart attack)

Physical symptoms of anxiety

- Racing pulse
- Sweating
- Clenching or grinding teeth
- Feeling breathless or unable to breathe deeply
- Feeling tight-chested
- Feeling light-headed
- Stomach upset or frequent bowel movements
- Feeling hot or flushed
- Lump in the throat
- Muscle tension
- Dry mouth
- Nausea
- Muscle weakness
- Fatigue
- Headache
- Loss of appetite

When anxiety persists it can impact in all areas of your life. You may begin to avoid doing the things that make you anxious which exacerbates the problem. Anxiety can be treated and I'll discuss the methods you can use in Part Three of the book.

Chapter Eighteen - Obsessive Compulsive Disorder (OCD)

The term OCD is often bandied about when talking about people who are 'neat freaks' or who clean a lot. While compulsive cleaning and tidiness is a trademark of OCD it is not the only symptom.

OCD is usually brought on by stress and anxiety, particularly during big life changes such as having a baby. People who suffer with OCD will experience unwelcome thoughts and urges, often followed by repetitive actions.

The obsessive nature of the illness focuses on persistent and uncontrollable thoughts, worries, fears or impulses which are very difficult to ignore.

The compulsive nature of the illness causes the person to carry out repetitive and persistent physical activities such as flicking light switches, checking and double checking locks on doors and can include mental thought rituals such as counting to a certain number before being able to fall asleep.

In my case, I had obsessive thoughts about germs in the atmosphere and in my food. These thoughts led me to carry out compulsive actions such as holding my breath when passing people in the street, frantically cleaning work surfaces before, during and after preparing food and washing my hands to the point that I would damage the skin.

With postnatal depression and anxiety, intrusive or obsessive thoughts on their own aren't a symptom of OCD. It is only when the person believes that something bad might happen, and that they will be responsible for this if they don't carry out certain rituals that OCD may be present. In more severe cases, OCD can result in self-harm, often unnoticed by the sufferer until afterwards (such as skin picking or scratching until they bleed).

OCD is seen as an anxiety disorder and many of the treatment methods will be similar and will be discussed in Part Three.

Chapter Nineteen - Birth Trauma/Post Traumatic Stress Disorder

Birth trauma occurs when a woman or her partner feels a severe threat to their lives or the lives or others (their baby or partner). This threat may be real, caused by actual events in the delivery room, or may be perceived threats, i.e. lives weren't actually in danger but the sufferer felt sufficiently frightened to perceive they were in danger. Birth trauma can occur even when a birth has been straightforward and uncomplicated. Birth trauma can be caused by a long or difficult labour and delivery, an unplanned caesarean section, emergency treatment or other unexpected events in the delivery room that led to the person feeling unsafe or vulnerable.

PTSD occurs when this trauma has a lasting and detrimental effect on the sufferer and can impede the person's ability to cope with every day tasks and impact their relationship with others, including the baby.

Symptoms of birth trauma/PTSD

- Flashbacks of the event
- Obsessively revisiting the event, playing it over and over, unable to move forward
- Intrusive thoughts and images
- Panic (usually triggered by some aspect of the event e.g. the smell of a hospital)
- Nightmares and disrupted sleep
- Intense distress at reminders of the trauma (real or perceived)
- Sweating, nausea, pain, numbness, trembling
- Outbursts of anger or irritability
- Hyper-alert for danger
- Lack of concentration
- Jumpiness or being easily startled
- Self-destructive behaviour or high-risk behaviour
- Avoiding situations that remind you of the event
- Numbing with alcohol or drugs
- Feelings of detachment, emotional numbness, not being able to connect with others
- Repressing memories
- Difficulty expressing affection or being vulnerable
- Unable to sit still, needing to be busy or distracted

PTSD is a very intense and distressing illness and yet is very treatable. We will explore treatment options in the next section of the book.

Chapter Twenty - Postnatal Psychosis

In contrast to the other mental illnesses postnatal psychosis is very rare, only occurring in around 1 in 1000 women after birth. It is a very serious condition that requires emergency medical treatment. Symptoms usually begin quite suddenly a few weeks, or in some cases days, after birth.

Symptoms of postnatal psychosis:

- Feeling excited or elated
- Rapid and extreme mood changes
- Feeling severely depressed
- Feeling confused or disorientated
- Feeling restless, unable to sleep or stop moving
- Unable to concentrate
- Experiencing hallucinations or delusions

Hallucinations and delusions

It's important to note the difference between delusions and hallucinations.

Hallucinations are when you see or hear things that aren't there. They can also appear as tastes, smells or sensations that you experience that others around you don't. You may hear voices or see people who aren't there. Usually the sufferer is unaware that they are experiencing anything unusual and don't realise they are ill until it is picked up by someone else.

Delusions are when you hold ideas or beliefs that others don't, such as having the ability to talk to God or control events such as the weather. They can include paranoia, thinking that someone is trying to harm you or your baby and it can be very distressing and intense.

No one really knows what causes postnatal psychosis but the the risks are raised if:

- You have bipolar disorder (this increases the risk of psychosis to one in four births)
- There is a history of mental illness in your family, particularly postnatal psychosis
- You have had a traumatic pregnancy or birth experience

Treatment

Treatment for postnatal psychosis will vary depending on the woman. In most cases you will be offered anti-psychotic medication and support from a mental health team. In more severe cases, you may need to be hospitalised, ideally in a mother and baby unit so that you are not separated from your baby. Very severe cases may require electroconvulsive therapy (ECT).

PART THREE:

TREATMENT

This section of the book will outline some of the tools, techniques and therapies which I, and many others have found helpful in our recovery. This is not an exhaustive list and not every technique will work for you. Try out those that appeal to you (or those that don't but that might help anyway!). Keep looking for other things that might work. Educating yourself about what's out there is your best way of finding the right fit for you.

You will find a list of resources to the back of the book that you can also access.

Chapter Twenty One - Self Help Techniques

This chapter will provide you with a selection of tips, tricks and techniques that you can try out yourself to help improve your mood, lower your stress levels and give you a toolkit that you can use whenever you need to in times of distress. This list isn't exhaustive but will give you a good place to start.

Breathing techniques

The breath is one of the most basic tools at our disposable. It can give us a point of focus, it can help bring us into the present moment instead of dwelling on the past or worrying about the future. It can help calm the nervous system in times of stress and anxiety. The beauty of breathing techniques is that you can do them anywhere. You don't need any special equipment and people around you don't necessarily have to know that you are doing them. Here are a few breathing techniques you can try out.

4-7-8 breath for relaxation

This breathing technique can be used to calm the body and bring about a state of relaxation. This exercise is very good for helping you to drift off to sleep or to bring calm after a period of anxiety or panic.

1. Place the tip of your tongue behind your upper front teeth and keep it there for the duration of the exercise.

2. With your mouth closed, inhale through your nose for a count of 4

3. Hold your breath for a count of 7

4. Purse your lips slightly and exhale through your mouth for a count of 8, making a slight 'whoosh' noise.

5. Repeat this cycle three more times.

Alternate Nostril Breathing

Taken from yoga, this breathing technique will help to energise and revitalise you. It is a good one to use first thing in the morning or during the afternoon slump. Many swear that it is as effective as a cup of coffee!

1. Sit in a comfortable upright position

2. Hold your right thumb against your right nostril, closing it completely but gently. Inhale slowly and deeply through the left nostril.

3. At the peak of inhalation, close the left nostril with your finger and exhale slowly through the right nostril.

4. Repeat the process, this time inhaling through the right nostril and exhaling through the left.

Diaphragmatic breathing for anxiety or panic

When a panic attack happens, the body begins to hyperventilate, increasing the level of oxygen in your blood stream to prepare the body for fight or flight. This reduces the level of carbon dioxide in your body. This breathing exercise focuses the breath back into a steady rhythm, balancing the levels of oxygen and carbon dioxide in your body. The trick is to breathe steadily but not too deeply. You may find some resistance from your body at the beginning of this exercise, after all it wants as much oxygen as possible and will give you an urge to take deep, fast breaths. Persevere and keep your breathing slow and steady. Eventually you will begin to feel more settled.

1. Sit up straight

2. Inhale slowly through your nose, breathing into your lower abdomen for a count of 4 (you can place a hand over your belly button while you practise. You should feel your belly rising as you inhale)

3. Hold your breath for a count of 2

4. Exhale slowly through your mouth for a count of 4

5. repeat as often as needed until the panic passes. Usually 6 to 8 cycles will be enough to settle panic.

Roll Breathing

This breathing technique will help you make full use of your lungs and to focus on the rhythm of your breathing. While learning, it's best to lie on your back with your knees up. Once you have mastered the skill you can do it anywhere.

1. Place your left hand on your lower abdomen and your right hand on your chest.

2. Inhale slowly through your nose, focusing the breath down into your lower belly. Your left hand should rise with the breath and the right hand should remain still. Exhale slowly through your mouth. Do this for 8 to 10 cycles.

3. When you have done this, begin again to inhale through your nose down into your lower belly and gradually allow the breath to fill the upper chest as well. When you exhale, make a slight whooshing noise with your mouth. Your left hand will begin to fall first, followed by your right hand.

4. Practice this technique for 3 to 5 minutes, noticing how your body begins to relax and release tension.

5. Practising this technique daily for several weeks will allow you to create a sense of instant relaxation wherever you are.

5-4-3-2-1 Exercise

To do this exercise, focus on your current environment and name:

5 things you can see

4 things you can feel (feet on the floor, a cool breeze...)

3 things you can hear

2 things you can smell (or things you like the smell of)

1 good thing about yourself

Pay attention to your senses and the details of those things you are naming.

Changing negative self-talk

1. Write down a list of the negative beliefs you hold about yourself, such as 'I'm not good enough'. Include any criticisms that others have made or that you perceive others to hold of you. Don't judge the statements as true or false. Simply write them down and notice how they make you feel in your body.

2. Now write down an affirmation to counter-act each of the negatives. Try to use words that are powerful. So for example, instead of 'I am good enough' you could say 'I am capable, worthy and an asset to my family'

3. Speak the affirmation out loud for 3 to 5 minutes, three times a day. You can do this while getting ready in the morning you can look at yourself in the mirror while you do it. Notice over time as your self-talk changes into something more pleasant.

Cognitive Awareness Exercise

Depression and anxiety can often lead to feelings of detachment and unreality. This exercise will help you to re-orient yourself in space and time by asking yourself some or all of these questions:

1. Where am I?

2. What is today?

3. What is the date?

4. What is the month?

5. What is the year?

6. How old am I?

7. What season is it?

Grounding Techniques

Grounding is the process of bringing your body and your awareness back into the present moment. It helps to keep you firmly in reality which is useful if you are prone to mulling over past events or worrying for the future. It can help regain focus with a sense of calm awareness.

Affirmations

Affirmations can seem like one of those airy-fairy techniques but don't be fooled. The brain is a powerful engine and language is vitally important in how the brain functions. Constant negative self-talk or worries show up in physical sensations and ailments in the body. It lowers our immune system and causes us to feel tired, ill and out of sorts. Positive affirmations can be used to change your mood and your state of mind.

Affirmations for mental health

- I am strong and capable
- I can handle anything that comes my way
- I am a good person, worthy of love
- I love myself for who I am
- I completely and totally accept myself
- I choose to let go of fear
- I choose to let go of anger
- How I feel is important
- I will come through this challenge stronger and more powerful
- I deserve to be happy
- I deserve to be loved
- I deserve to be supported
- My body and my mind are worthy of care
- I can express my thoughts and feelings without fear or judgment
- I trust in my ability to get better
- I am safe, I am calm, I am relaxed

You can add to this list any affirmations that work for you. Affirmations are a very personal thing so choose those that feel right for you and practise every day.

Mindfulness & Meditation

Mindfulness is a mental state achieved by focusing awareness on the present moment while calmly acknowledging and accepting one's feelings, thoughts and bodily sensations. Mindfulness is similar to grounding in that it brings the body and the mind into the present moment. This can feel uncomfortable at first but with daily practice it quickly becomes more natural. Research indicates that mindfulness and meditation can be effective treatments for a range of mental illnesses. It not only helps us to feel more calm and grounded, it actually changes the structure and wiring of the brain, leading to a calmer and more relaxed state when practised regularly.

Simple mindfulness meditation practice

1. Find somewhere comfortable to sit upright where it is quiet and free from distractions

2. With your eyes open and with soft focus, take five slow, deep breaths, inhaling through the nose and exhaling through the mouth. On the final exhale, slowly allow your eyes to close. Allow your breathing pattern to return to normal.

3. Beginning at the top of your head, slowly scan down through your body, noting any areas of tension or relaxation. Don't aim to change these, just notice them in the body.

4. Bring your attention back to the breath. Notice where you feel the breath in the body, the cool air in your nostrils, the rise and fall of your abdomen. If it helps, you can count the breath, inhale 1, exhale 2, inhale 3 etc... Once you reach 10 start again at 1. If you lose track, just begin again at 1.

5. It's perfectly natural for the mind to wander. If you notice this happening, gently bring the attention back to the breath. Continue this way for 5 minutes.

6. When it's time to stop, become more aware of your surroundings, the sounds you hear, the feel of your body in the chair. Slowly open your eyes and take a moment to notice how you feel. Are you more relaxed? Calmer?

The Resources section has more ideas for meditation support.

Paradoxical Intention for Panic Attacks

This is one of those techniques that feels completely counter-intuitive and will make you want to run a mile, and yet it works so well.

When you've been taken over by a panic attack, your brain is doing precisely what we don't want it to do, over-reacting to a perceived threat. Paradoxical intention works to reduce the anxiety by inviting the brain to make the reaction even stronger, more intense, more panicky. By doing this, you are bringing all of those intense sensations under voluntary control, thus accepting your symptoms and allowing them to exist. The message this sends to your fight-or-flight response is that you have the situation under control and it can stand down.

How to use paradoxical intention during a panic attack

1. Use the diaphragmatic breathing exercise at the beginning of this chapter to regulate your breathing

2. Don't fight the symptoms of your panic or escape to your safe space

3. Acknowledge the most intense sensation you are feeling right now (heart racing, sweating etc.)

4. Say to yourself: "I am taking control of this sensation. I would like (my heart to race faster)(to sweat more)"

5. Consciously attempt to increase the intensity of that symptom

6. Now do this for all the symptoms (nausea, dizziness etc). "Let's see if I can make my legs turn to jelly right now).

7. Keep breathing steadily while you do this.

8. Try to avoid thoughts of 'this isn't working'. Keep your focus on what you are doing and the symptoms will resolve.

This is a difficult technique to master since the only time you can practise it is when you are in full-scale panic mode. It really works though so bear it in mind!

Emotional Freedom Technique (EFT)/Tapping

EFT is a technique which helps release negative emotion by tapping on various meridian energy points on the body. I have to admit I was sceptical about this one but after five minutes of tapping during a pretty intense panic attack, I was overcome by a feeling of calm, to the point that I almost felt 'zoned out'. I'm a total convert and use this when faced with any situation that makes me anxious such as flying or before a job interview.

The technique is quite difficult to explain on paper so I've included a few links to videos and demonstrations in the Resources section for you check out.

Self Care and Compassion

One of the simplest things we can do for our mental health is to look after ourselves, and yet self-care is usually the first to go out the window when our mental health takes a dip. It can also be difficult with children, a job, a household to run, a marriage to maintain and all the other little things that get in the way during the course of our day. However, self-care doesn't need to be a major activity that requires planning and effort. Often it's the small things that make the most difference. For me, it is a bath after the kids have gone to bed, just thirty minutes with no noise, no phone and no interruptions, just time to be.

Self-care works best when you incorporate it into your routine. This could mean getting up twenty minutes before every one else to have a cup of tea in the quiet before starting your day. It could be a walk after dinner or a ten minute meditation practice. Keeping your self-care routine simple will make it easier to become a habit in your life. It can also be helpful to create a list of things you can do in five minutes, fifteen minutes, thirty minutes etc. so that if you find yourself with a chunk of time free, you can quickly find something that nourishes you.

Here are a few examples to get you started:

Five minutes or less:

- Smell your favourite scent
- Play your favourite song
- Dance around the kitchen
- Step outside and take big breath of fresh air
- Have a snack
- Write down your thoughts
- Massage some essential oils into your wrists or temples
- Call a friend for a chat
- Check out a five minute meditation on YouTube

Fifteen minutes

- Have a cup of tea
- Grab a hot shower
- Do a crossword/sudoku
- Take a walk outside
- Meditate
- Give yourself a facial
- Read a chapter of a book
- Watch an uplifting TED Talk
- Cuddle with your partner
- Do some light exercise
- Disconnect from technology and just sit in the quiet

Thirty minutes

- Have a soak in the bath

- Book a massage

- Go for a coffee with a friend

- Do something creative (draw, write, knit)

- Take a nap

- Take a class/hobby

- Go shopping/to the library/anywhere that makes you happy

- Get out into nature

- Take a drive and listen to your favourite band

Self-Compassion

One of the biggest problems we face when we suffer with a mental illness is the seemingly unending negative chatter inside our heads. We tell ourselves we are weak or unworthy, we berate ourselves for not being stronger, we blame ourselves for the position we find ourselves in. This is the illness talking. When we catch a cold, we feel miserable but we don't spend our days telling ourselves how stupid we were to have caught the cold. It's ridiculous, and yet when we are ill in our mind we lose all sense of compassion and caring for ourselves.

There is no one to blame for mental illness, it just is. The best way to fight it is to become friends with it, and with ourselves. By becoming patient and compassionate with ourselves, we get a greater understanding of ourselves and of others. We become more empathic and connected to those around us and we are better able to see the illness for what it truly is.

How can we be more self-compassionate? Firstly we need to thank our inner demons for trying to protect us. That is, in part, what's happening after all. Our brains are telling us that the outside world is a scary and difficult place to be. That it is better to be cut off and not be hurt than to be vulnerable and risk humiliation, further pain or worse. Try to change that inner voice from one of judgment to one of empathy. Say:

"Thank you brain for trying to take care of me, but I can handle this."

When you catch a thought such as 'I am worthless', use the affirmations at the beginning of this chapter to counter it with a self-compassionate phrase, 'I am worthy of love, respect and support'.

Don't allow the illness to isolate you. Find people that you can connect with. Mental illness can only thrive in the lonely dark. Shine a light on it and find someone you can trust to share with. This is not a fight that anyone should have to go through alone. Community, connection and friendship will serve you well in your recovery.

Be your own best friend also. Try to see your thoughts and your illness from an outsider's perspective. Imagine a friend or relative in your situation. What would you say to them? How would you comfort them? What advice would you give? Do that for yourself.

Chapter Twenty Two - Talking Therapies

Talking is one of the most effective ways to explore our thoughts and feelings and build connections with those around us. Talking therapies involve speaking with a trained professional about your worries and issues, exploring ways in which you can address these and to practice coping strategies and techniques to improve your mental health. While talking to a friend or family member can provide relief from your distress, a trained professional can help you to go deeper and can help you manage your thoughts and emotions in a safe space. It also helps to have someone impartial to share your thoughts with without worrying about hurting anyone's feelings or causing upset.

There are a range of talking therapies available through the NHS, privately and through voluntary bodies. It might take a while to find the type of therapy or the therapist that works for you but when you find it, marvellous things can happen. Outlined below are just a few of the types of talking therapies available.

Cognitive Behavioural Therapy (CBT)

CBT is a practical and scientific way to examine your thoughts and emotions, helping you to understand how these thoughts and feelings arise. It uses practical tools to manage the symptoms of distress. For example, by understanding the cycle of a panic attack, you can use tools to interrupt the cycle and bring yourself back to a place of calm.

While a CBT therapist will help you explore the root cause of your issues, the focus is very much on the here and now, using practical tools and coping strategies. It can be very effective, particularly for anxiety and panic. Treatment is usually short term, between six and twenty four sessions with a therapist. This type of therapy will suit anyone who is goal-driven and likes to have a structured plan they can follow.

Provision of CBT through the NHS can be patchy and usually has long waiting lists so private treatment might be an option for you. If this is the case, be sure to research any potential therapist, making sure they have the appropriate qualifications and experience.

Interpersonal Psychotherapy for Depression (IPT)

IPT is growing in popularity as an effective treatment for postnatal depression. Like CBT, it is a short-term therapy usually lasting twelve to sixteen weeks and aims to reduce the severity of symptoms and puts in place coping strategies. The focus of IPT is to build connections between the client and his or her support network, thus creating stronger bonds, a more robust support system and increased confidence. IPT for postnatal depression looks at the life changes and transition of having a new baby as causes of the depression as well as friction in close relationships and the sense of loss that a parent can feel when a baby is born (such as the loss of identity). IPT follows a manual and is very structured and goal-orientated.

Rewind Therapy

Rewind therapy is used to settle the distress surrounding birth trauma or post-traumatic stress disorder (PTSD). Rewind therapy is very effective at helping the parent process birth trauma in as little as two to three sessions. The treatment involves three steps:

1. Retelling the story of the trauma (this does not have to be done out loud, but it does need to be remembered to be understood), and understanding how you would like to feel after the therapy

2. Going into a state of deep relaxation and exploring the trauma in a safe and secure way

3. Using your imagination to see what life can be like without the traumatic symptoms.

While this seems incredibly simplistic, it works on a neurological level, helping the brain to process the traumatic memories and settling down the body's 'alarm system' so it isn't triggered, allowing you to live your life without the trauma resurfacing time and again.

Counselling

Counselling can differ from the talking therapies above in that it is not a time-limited, structured therapy. Rather, a counsellor is there to provide a safe and confidential environment for you to talk through your problems, identify the causes and explore your specific ways of thinking. A counsellor is not there to provide solutions but can guide you through your own thought processes to find a way out of your distress. Counselling can be very effective in treating ante- and post-natal mental illness by helping you comes to terms with the changes happening in your life and finding ways to cope more effectively.

Eye Movement Desensitisation and Reprocessing (EMDR)

EMDR is used to treat trauma and needs to be carried out by a trained specialist. When we experience a trauma, the traumatic memory is either stored in the left side of our brain (the logical side) or the right side of our brain (the emotional side). Using EMDR, the parent recalls the traumatic experience while following the movement of the clinician's finger. This allows both sides of the brain to communicate and integrate, processing the memories more effectively which reduces the intensity of the memories over time.

Psychiatry

In the more extreme cases of severe depression or psychosis, it is vital that the parent is seen by a trained psychiatrist, particularly with postnatal psychosis as this is considered a medical emergency. Psychiatric treatment will vary by patient but will usually take the form of a combination of medication and talking therapy. In the most difficult cases, this may require inpatient treatment at a specialist unit. Evidence shows that keeping the mother and baby together during this stay is a vital component of recovery and mother-infant bonding and is therefore the best solution for the mother to be admitted to a specialist mother and baby unit. Unfortunately in the UK, these are few and far between and many parents are separated from their babies at this time while they receive this vital treatment. If you or someone you love requires inpatient care, find out if there is a mother and baby unit in your area. If not, discuss your options with your care-giver to see if there is a way they can accommodate optimal contact between the mother and baby.

Wellness Recovery Action Plan® (WRAP®)

The Wellness Recovery Action Plan® is a document that you can create yourself that will help you identify your triggers, what support you might need at any given time and a toolkit for getting you from a place of despair to a place of wellness. It is a great resource for both the person suffering with mental illness and their supporters as it gives a clear step-by-step process for managing a variety of situations, including a crisis plan in case you find yourself in crisis. You can find a link to the WRAP® information in the Resources section.

Chapter Twenty Three - Medication

I didn't want to write this book and avoid the topic of medication. That said, I am definitely not an expert in this subject and also don't want to steer you down the wrong path. What I have provided here is a brief description of the types of medication used to treat mental illness in parents. Please remember that all medications should be taken only on the advice of a medical professional. If you feel that medication is right for you, please consult your doctor for guidance and be sure to also let them know if you are pregnant or breastfeeding.

Antidepressants

There are a range of antidepressants available that work in different ways. They are recommended for moderate to severe depression or anxiety, usually in conjunction with talking therapy. They work by balancing the chemicals in the brain which can ease symptoms such as low mood, irritability and lack of concentration. They usually need to be taken for a few weeks before the benefits can be felt. There may be a number of side effects which usually settle after a few weeks but it is important to discuss these with your doctor if you are experiencing any unwanted symptoms. It is also worth considering if the benefits of the medication outweigh the impact of the side effects, which can include:

- Nausea
- Blurred vision
- Dry mouth
- Constipation
- Dizziness or fogginess
- Feeling shaky
- Feeling agitated
- Low sex drive
- Feelings of emotional numbness or disconnect

Anxiolytics

Anxiolytics are a group of medicines used to treat anxiety disorders. They tend to work very quickly and can be habit-forming, therefore they are usually only prescribed in the short-term. They are often sedative in nature and can cause drowsiness which may impact on daily activities. These are usually prescribed in conjunction with therapy such a CBT. Anxiolytics range from antidepressants, antihistamines and benzodiazepines, all of which target the chemicals in the body that create and sustain states of anxiety and panic. Again, there are side effects including:

- Drowsiness
- Digestive upset
- Confusion
- Sexual dysfunction
- Headache
- Suicidal thoughts
- High blood pressure
- Weight gain

Beta Blockers

Beta blockers are traditionally used to treat heart conditions such as angina and high blood pressure, however they are often prescribed to treat anxiety. They work by blocking the effects of norepinephrine (the stress hormone involved in panic and anxiety) thus reducing the physical sensations of anxiety. While it doesn't impact the emotional symptoms of anxiety such as worry or negative thoughts, it may provide some relief from the physical symptoms, allowing the person some space to process their emotions. They are short-lived medications, usually out of the system within twelve hours and are often used to manage phobias such as flying or performance anxiety. Like all medications, they also may have some side effects such as:

- Dizziness
- Drowsiness
- Weakness
- Fatigue

- Nausea
- Headache
- Constipation
- Diarrhoea

Supplements

While the effectiveness of taking supplements has not been conclusively proven, many swear by the effects of supplements and many doctors now offer these as a prescription.

B Vitamins such as B6, B9 and B12 are known to convert tryptophan into serotonin. Low levels of zinc and iron have also been linked to depression and therefore taking a supplement may help reduce symptoms.

St John's Wort is used regularly to treat depression as it is thought to increase levels of serotonin in the body. Be very careful if you are already taking an antidepressant and this can cause serotonin poisoning, a very dangerous medical condition.

Chapter Twenty Four - Physical Wellbeing

Much like self-care, when we begin to feel anxious or depressed we stop doing the things that are key to helping us feel better. Low energy and motivation often leads to poor choices for our bodies and can really impact on our body's ability to recover. With Western medicine there has been a long history of treating the mind and the body as two separate entities. The latest research is showing that actually, the two are inextricably linked and to provide the best care, we need to treat the whole person, not individual parts of the person.

One of the best ways you can help your recovery is to ensure that you are putting as much effort into looking after your body as you are your mind.

Diet

We already know that low levels of iron and zinc are linked to depression but there are other aspects of our diet that need to be taken into consideration as well. There is growing research on the link between our gut and our central nervous system (known as the gut-brain axis or GBA). In fact, the gut is now being seen as a second 'brain' and both brains communicate to each other in both directions. This explains that 'gut-wrenching' feeling we get when we are anxious. A study done in 2017 has shown that sensitivity to gut stimuli influences our brain in a perpetual feedback loop and affects our moods, frame of mind, and how we perceive the world around us. This works both ways as anyone who has had a panic attack will testify. Emotional triggers can set off a range of intestinal issues such as diarrhoea, cramping and nausea.

In order to keep the body balanced and both 'brains' functioning at optimum levels we need to address not only the emotional triggers, but the physical triggers as well. The way to do this is to balance the flora in the gut by managing your diet. Did you know that serotonin, the 'happy' hormone is stored mainly in the gut? Low levels of serotonin have long been connected to depression. Over 90% of serotonin is found in the gut with only 5-10% found in the brain. Therefore it makes sense to eat foods that can promote healthy gut flora and boost serotonin production. To give you an idea of how mainstream this thinking is becoming, many mental health professionals are now regularly prescribing probiotics as part of treatment plans for their patients with mental illness.

So how can you change your diet to improve your mood? First off, I would recommend that before you start any diet or exercise programme, you speak to your doctor to ensure there are no health reasons why you shouldn't. If you have the all clear, then you can try some of the below:

Just eat real food (JERF)

JERF diets such as paleo have be growing in popularity over the past few years. The basic premise is to cut out all foods that have been processed or refined and eat as our ancestors did, fresh fruit, vegetables and meat. There are some links in the Resources section for more information but to give you an idea, here are the things you would cut from your diet:

- Refined sugar
- Dairy products
- Grains, pulses and beans
- Bread
- Nightshades such as white potatoes
- Caffeine

Now I know you have just looked at that list and thought, what can I eat!? You will be surprised with how many of these things you can happily live without with a few substitutions. For example, you can replace sugar with raw honey.

I tried a paleo diet for six weeks when I was in the worst stages of anxiety and depression and it made a huge difference. The first week was pretty horrendous as my body adjusted to meals that weren't loaded with bread and stodgy food but once that had settled, I found myself with energy to burn and for those six weeks I felt better than I have in years. I felt like I could run a marathon and didn't suffer a single panic attack or have any anxiety the whole time.

If it's so great, why didn't I stick to it? It is not an easy plan to follow if you value convenience or if you are on a tight budget, which let's face it, is the case for most families with young children. All food is prepared fresh, it's difficult to find a quick snack and sometimes you really just NEED the bread. If you have the time and resources, give it a go.

Serotonin-boosting foods

Add more of these foods into your diet to boost serotonin production:

Fermented foods such as kefir, sauerkraut, kimchi, kombucha, cultured vegetable juices and jun tea. These are probiotic and will help balance your gut flora and aid in the digestion of the nutrients we need to process and absorb serotonin

Vitamin B6

This is another supplement that GPs are regularly prescribing for conditions such as depression, PMS and anxiety. Eat these foods to get your daily dose:

- Cauliflower
- Fish
- Spinach
- Mushrooms
- Celery
- Eggs
- Garlic
- Chicken
- Beef

Eggs are also high in tryptophan, the amino acid from which serotonin is derived.

It goes without saying that takeaways, sugar, alcohol and junk food are going to have a detrimental effect on your physical and mental health. Too much sugar is stimulating and can exacerbate feelings of restlessness, anxiety and agitation as well as interrupting sleep. A little bit of chocolate can be beneficial for serotonin production so it's not all bad news!

Exercise

If you're like me, the thought of exercise makes you groan, and not in a good way! If you suffer with a panic disorder, the physical sensations associated with exercise (increased heart rate, sweating) can be enough to trigger an attack and so you might avoid exercise like the plague.

If there is no physical reason for you not to exercise, this can be one of most useful tools in your toolkit.

Being outside, particularly in green spaces has been shown to have a marked effect on mood and mental health. Exercise helps our bodies to use up all those stress hormones that have been flooding our systems as a result of stress. It doesn't need to be strenuous exercise either. A brisk walk, going up and down the stairs, even dancing around your bedroom all count.

Exercise is particularly important if you have recently had a panic attack. Your body will be prepped and ready for action and the best way to settle those feelings is through movement. By allowing your muscles to use up those stress hormones, you allow your nervous system to reset itself and go back to a state of rest.

Sleep

One of the most difficult experiences about becoming a new parent is adjusting to the frequent and very normal night wakings of a baby. There is a whole industry out there making billions of pounds selling sleep aids to tired parents, promising them nights of unbroken sleep like they had before the baby was born. I call bullshit. You may strike lucky and get one of those babies who sleeps twelve hours straight from day one. I had one of those. I also had two babies who woke every hour, on the hour and screamed bloody murder, driving me to distraction for months on end. What I discovered with my third baby (a night-owl) is that for my own mental health, the best thing to do was roll with it, don't fight it. Accept that that's just how it is for now and it won't be forever. Does that mean there weren't nights when I wanted to leave her on the doorstep? No, I struggled plenty. What it did do was relieve me from all this pressure of how my baby 'should' be sleeping.

Aside from an active baby, mental illness also causes disruption in sleep. There is nothing more cruel than finally collapsing into bed exhausted after a long day's struggle only to find that your brain has gone into overdrive and try as you might you can't sleep. Or you might be like me and be able to fall asleep fine only to be woken mid-panic, drenched in sweat and struggling to breathe.

When your sleep suffers, it impacts every other part of your life. You become irritable, fatigued and lose interest in things that usually make you happy. You struggle to hold conversations or concentrate on anything for extended periods of time. It also just makes you feel simply rotten.

What can you do to help improve your sleep? Any of the techniques below may help you regain control over your sleep routine. Try any or all of them, add more to the list if you come across something that helps:

- Switch off electronics at least an hour before bedtime. Blue light from TV screens, phones and computers stimulate the brain. Not what you need before bed!

- Engage in calming activity before bed such as taking a bath, reading a book or meditating

- Listen to a self-hypnosis track

- Listen to an audiobook or podcast (the calmer the better, you don't need to be listening to a horror story just as you're drifting off!)

- If you have a partner, ask for a back rub/foot rub using lavender oil which is known for its relaxing properties

- Don't nap during the day unless you have had a really long night and really must. Napping can interrupt your natural sleeping pattern and make it difficult to sleep later

- Create a routine: get up at the same time every day and go to bed at the same time every night. Just like we do with children, create a set of sleep cues that your brain can pick up on to prepare you for sleep. My routine is usually to have a bath, read a chapter of a book and switch on an audiobook. By the time the audiobook is on, my body is ready for sleep and I barely last 3 minutes (thank goodness for the sleep timer!)

- Try the 4-7-8 breathing technique outlined earlier in the book

- If none of this is working, speak to your GP about medication.

Epsom Salts

One thing that I have found very helpful is Epsom salts (or magnesium sulphate) in the bath. We know that stress, anxiety and insomnia release cortisol, adrenaline and epinephrine into the body, all of which depletes magnesium levels. Guess what happens when your magnesium levels are low? That's right, you get anxious.

Magnesium is difficult to get from your diet, especially as you also need Vitamin D for your body to process it. Taking a supplement orally can increase your magnesium levels but may cause some unwanted effects on your digestive system. Studies have shown that the best way to absorb magnesium is through your skin.

Adding one or two cups of Epsom salts to a warm bath and soaking for at least twelve minutes can increase your magnesium levels and reduce anxiety. It also relaxes the muscles (try it after a workout!) and a soak in the bath is soothing for the mind.

I was sceptical when I first began using Epsom salts a few years ago. The effect was so marked that I began to wonder if I had an anxiety disorder at all or whether I was just magnesium-deficient! I now bulk buy and never let them run out. I have an Epsom salts bath at least twice a week with a few drops of lavender oil in the water and it's absolute bliss.

Chapter Twenty Five - Social Support

One of the biggest protective factors for mental health is strong interpersonal relationships, having someone to talk to about your worries and who can support you through the difficult times. Unfortunately, with the rise of technology and social media, we are losing our communities and becoming more isolated and withdrawn.

While we are more connected than ever, with hundreds of 'friends' on social media right across the world, we are also more insular. We share images of the things that are going well in our lives and rarely share the uglier side of our lives. We filter our Instagram photos to blur out our imperfections and we all appear to be living our 'best lives'. Is this really the case? We are bombarded with images from others and compare our lives to those picture perfect moments we see others sharing several times a day. It is no wonder that when life becomes hard, we find it difficult to open up. Especially given that much of our interactions these days seem to take place through the medium of an electronic device, it can seem almost impossible find the words we need to share our distress.

So what can we do about it? One of the biggest changes you can make in your life when you are suffering from a mental illness is to identify your support network and reach out for help. This can be incredibly unsettling, especially when mental illness will make you want to withdraw from contact and isolate yourself. This is the ideal environment for mental illness to thrive and it will drain your energy, your motivation and your desire to connect with others because that's how it survives.

Connecting with others, getting those dark, scary or downright irrational thoughts out of your head by speaking them out loud to a trusted supporter can make all the difference. It will help those thoughts seem less powerful and help you gain an insight into how you can manage them.

When you feel heard and felt by someone else, it also helps you to feel less alone. Loneliness is one of the most damaging experiences a human being can go through, both mentally and physically. When we feel alone, our immune system lowers, stress levels increase and we can become physically and chronically ill if it is not addressed.

So how do you improve your social support? Some of you will already have a good network of friends or family that you can access. Find someone you trust and talk to them about how you're feeling. Allow yourself to be vulnerable and speak candidly about what is going on for you. Make a point to see your friends and family on a regular and consistent basis if you can. This doesn't always have to be to talk about how you're feeling. Sometimes just doing something nice with someone is enough to lift your mood, help you feel more connected and strengthen your bonds.

Not everyone will have a strong support network or a trusted person to talk to. In that instance, seek out others in the same situation. You can join a support group, find a hobby that you enjoy and can meet new people or volunteer with a local charity. This can also help to boost your self-esteem by doing something good for others while building your confidence as you learn new skills.

The key here is to be brave. When you see an opportunity to engage with someone, rather than shying away, participate! You can make the most unlikely and best of friends by opening yourself up to new experiences. Sometimes all it takes is to say hello to someone to begin a beautiful friendship.

Social prescribing

Social prescribing is becoming more common within the NHS whereby GPs are able to refer their patients to services in the community rather than solely providing a medicalised solution. The GP refers the patient to a 'community connector' who can talk to the person, find out about the things that are important to them and together, create a social prescription that will help improve their wellbeing.

Activities that people can be prescribed can range from art classes to choirs, running clubs, gardening groups and cookery classes. These activities help to bring people together, break down isolation, reduce loneliness and help build a stronger community of supportive individuals.

Not only is social prescribing helping with the health and wellbeing of patients, it is also reducing the number of people visiting their GP or A&E departments, reducing use of medication and the likelihood of being referred to social care.

You might be asking yourself if going to an art class or singing in a choir will really make that much difference to your mental health. An evidence-led study by the University of Westminster suggests that it really does have an impact. And what do you have to lose?

Chapter Twenty Six - Conclusion

It has been a long six years as I have struggled with my mental health. At times the road was only slightly bumpy, at other times it felt so steep and rocky that I doubted my own ability to walk it. The start of parenthood for me was fraught with uncertainty, worry and unbelievable stress. It was not the magical fairytale I imagined it would be. I will always mourn the fact that I missed out on so much joy with my babies because of this horrible illness.

My journey with perinatal mental illness isn't over yet, I still have days where I struggle with anxiety, occasional panic attacks and low moods. What has changed is that I no longer feel so confined and weighed down by my illness. I am able to see it for what it is, a disorganisation of my mind and a response to many years of being in survival mode. I hold out hope that in the near future, I will once again visit the seaside and be able to breathe freely and let the anxiety and stress fall away and be at peace. I'm choosing to focus on a brighter future.

Don't get me wrong, during the more difficult days it can feel impossible to see a life without mental illness, but on those days I remind myself of all the days I had before, free from it's grip, and I work on it using the toolkit I've developed over these past few years to give myself the best shot. Then I wait it out. It is also important to remember that bad days are sometimes just that...bad days. It doesn't always mean that I am sliding back down the rabbit hole or spiralling out of control. One of the meanest aspects of mental illness is that it can make the everyday difficult times feel like the beginning of a downward spiral. It's easy to let this assumption take over and bring you back to the bad place. Or you can choose to recognise that this is just a bad day and it will pass like all the other bad days have passed. It's important also to recognise that your perspective might be off. I remember a period when my eldest was young, thinking that every day for months was horrendous and I couldn't remember a single positive thing that happened. When I reread my journal from that time recently, I realised that actually, the bad days weren't every day. Sometimes they weren't even most of one week. There were stretches of good days when I felt lighter and easier but my focus on the bad times completely coloured out the good and made me think that the torment was unending. It wasn't. I'm working now to try to remember the better moments of those early days and reclaim some of the joy I lost with my daughter.

If you take anything away from this book, I think I would like it to be this: connection is everything. The only way to fully recover is to find meaningful connections to those around you, to yourself, to your work. We can't weather the storm of mental illness alone. Medication, therapy and self-help practices will all serve you well to improve your mental health and get you to a more stable, less reactive place in your life and you can live very well using these alone but people...people are what make our lives nourishing and worthwhile. If you don't have a support network, find one. Don't listen to those inner demons telling you that you aren't worthy, or good enough, or smart enough or funny enough. Don't let your illness tell you that you don't have the energy or motivation. That is how the illness keeps you down. You need more than ever to find your fight, stand up and reclaim your life. Not just for your sake but also for your family and for your children.

Anxiety and depression have robbed me of many precious moments in my life. I have turned down opportunities, deprived myself of experiences that would have enriched my life and most of all, made me feel that I was failing. Failing myself and failing my husband and children. I am so grateful that I found my fight and was able recognise the lies my illness told me. My children, who I love more than anything in the world, get to have a better mother and a better childhood because I found my fight.

It seems counter-intuitive but I am also grateful for the journey I have been on over the last six years. Not only has it made me stronger and more resilient, it has made me more compassionate towards others and more understanding of the motivations of other people. Now when I see someone acting out, I can clearly see the hurt behind the behaviour and can empathise with that person so much better. This allows me, not only to respond in a compassionate and constructive way, it also allows me to maintain my own equilibrium when faced with these challenging circumstances. I no longer take other people's reactions personally (or at least I try not to!).

Because of my struggle with my own mental health I have become an expert by lived experience. I have researched such a range of techniques and therapies that my survival toolkit is well-stocked and serves me well. It also helps me to help my children. My eldest daughter Alexis struggles with anxiety and worries about her health and mortality. It breaks my heart to know she has picked up much of this from me despite my best efforts to shield her from it. It also means that I am able to teach her tools to manage her own mental health. Our family is very aware of how important looking after our mental wellbeing is and by having this open dialogue, we hope to be able to build more resilient children. By teaching them the tools that I have discovered through my own struggle, I hope to prepare them for when they face their own difficulties later in life.

My struggle has also helped me to understand my parents much better and to appreciate the impossible situation they were in when we were growing up. Dealing with their own issues, the immense pressure they were under and trying to give us the best childhood was an unimaginable task. Now that I have an insight into how they struggled when we were children, I can empathise and view my own childhood experiences through a new lens. Many of the things that made me feel slighted or wronged and that dogged me for years can now be let go. I can see how fortunate I am to have parents who despite all the challenges they faced, managed to give me a childhood full of happy memories and an adulthood that I can be proud of.

I have discovered something recently that is proving to be one of the most healing and joyous experiences. Now that my children are old enough to play and make believe, I find myself revisiting moments from my own childhood and seeing it through their eyes. It is almost as though I can relive all those small but significant moments that I found so much pleasure in and that I had forgotten about through all the busyness of adulthood. Playing with Lego, putting on a puppet show or a dance recital. Bandaging dollies, climbing fences, learning to tumble. The questions and curiosity and the love for animals. These are all the things that made my own childhood so special and through my children, I have been able to shift my focus from a terrible thing that happened to me as a young girl, and relive my childhood once more without the panic and stress and worry of carrying around a mammoth secret. It has also focused my attention on my own children and how important it is to enjoy them while they are little. I heard a phrase when Alexis was a small baby:

"You will never be as loved as you are now."

It is so true. As they grow and become more dependent, as they find partners of their own and go out into the world, they will never be as close or as in love with their mother as they are right now. I don't want mental illness to rob me of this experience like it has so many others. I want to be able to look back on this time and say that even when it was hard, and exhausting, and mundane, that I relished it as much as I could, and to have no regrets.

I think it is also important to note that the attitude our society has towards mental illness needs to drastically change. We view mental illness as this scary, shameful and awkward illness that needs to be hidden away. We judge those with mental illness as though they are making a choice to be ill, that they would feel better if they adjusted their attitude. This is absolutely not the case. I have often felt extremely frustrated when the logical side of my brain is completely aware of how the illness was affecting me and yet feeling totally powerless to change it. Mental illness is not a choice.

We need to start treating it like any other illness, with compassion, care and understanding. We need to open the dialogue with our friends and loved ones, to have candid conversations about our wellbeing, the same way we do about our physical ailments. We need to hold those suffering and find a way to support them without judgment or criticism. We need better services to diagnose and treat mental illnesses quickly and fully.

We are facing an epidemic of mental illness all across the world, and the effects are long ranging. They don't just have an impact on the sufferer but on their partners, their children and their wider communities for years to follow. It is not good enough that people who are feeling suicidal or at risk are having to wait months on referrals or assistance. It is not good enough to say that those who die from a mental illness are simply taking the coward's way out. Suicide is not a choice. It is a lack of choice. Depression and anxiety can make your life feel so utterly unbearable that although you don't want to die, it feels like the only way to relieve the pain. It is a symptom of mental illness. It is a succumbing to mental illness, that same way that some people succumb to cancer or pneumonia or heart failure. It is not a choice and we need to stop looking at it like it is.

When it comes to parents in particular, having a baby is one of the most monumental and life-changing transitions that a person can go through and yet it is the one we are least prepared for. We spend thirteen years in school preparing us for work, we learn from our families how to manage money, keep a household, do the grocery shopping. If we want to take a holiday we research, educate ourselves and save. When it comes to preparing for a baby, we are not doing enough to prepare parents. We have our standard antenatal classes that look at labour, pain relief, car seat safety but we do very little to prepare parents not just for the physical aftermath of childbirth (pain, sleep disruption, even being able to sit down to a meal) but for the emotional aftermath. No one is telling parents how to look after their mental wellbeing during one of the most stressful and important times in their lives. Even if we don't take mental illness into consideration, parents are still struggling to manage their moods, their temper and their relationships when faced with the pressures of looking after a tiny human.

We are not providing new parents with the skills and techniques to help ease them into parenthood and navigate this uncertain and challenging time. When we do take mental illness into consideration, not only are we not doing enough to educate parents on the potential difficulties they may face, we are also not doing enough to support them when they occur. Why is it that this most important job, raising children, has become so under-valued? Why are we so dismissive of the needs of new parents who are struggling? We need to do more, and to do it NOW. The future generations depend on it.

A healthy population begins with healthy parents who are able to raise healthy and well-adjusted children. That is not just the job of the parents themselves, but the wider community to support and guide them. We need to bring back our village and take responsibility for the collective health and wellbeing of everyone in our community. So put down your phone, close your social media and engage with those around you. If you find someone who is struggling, find a way to help. Educate yourself on ways to be a great supporter. Ask questions, be free to chat when you can, see if there is something practical you can do to help out parents who are struggling (send round a dinner, do a load of laundry). Make the conversation about mental wellbeing a regular one in your household and help to end the stigma that so many people are struggling with today.

I hope that you found this book helpful for whatever stage of your journey you are on. It is my sincerest wish that you or your loved one makes a full and speedy recovery from this illness and that you move on to a life that is as full and as beautiful as you deserve. Thank you for sharing this experience and I wish you every success.

Resources

Here you will find links to all the resources mentioned in this book. I hope you find these useful and insightful. This is not an exhaustive list and new resources are being developed every day. This is a good starting point for you to begin to find the tools you need to begin and sustain your recovery.

Websites

PANGS

An online resource site for all things related to perinatal mental illness.

www.wearepangs.com

NI Maternal Mental Health Conference

A Northern Ireland based conference which brings together parents, professionals and volunteers to explore ways to improve services for women and their families

www.maternalmentalhealth.co.uk

NI Positive Birth Conference

A Northern Ireland based conference aimed at educating and promoting positive birth experiences for all parents

www.positivebirthconference.co.uk

Moment Health

An app which parents can download to track their symptoms, check their moods and find out how to seek additional support

www.momenthealth.io

NCT Hidden Half

A campaign to demand better six-week postnatal check-ups so that all new mothers with a mental health problem can access the treatment available.

www.nct.org.uk/get-involved/campaigns/hidden-half

NCT Parents in Mind

Parents in Mind is a peer support model that trains local volunteers to support women experiencing emotional health difficulties in pregnancy and the first two years after birth.

www.nct.org.uk/professional/parents-in-mind

Have You Seen That Girl?

Blogger and campaigner Lindsay Robinson shares her own, and others' stories of perinatal mental illness as well as campaigning for better services in Northern Ireland.

www.haveyouseenthatgirl.com

Olivia Siegl (Every Mum Movement/Bonkers)

Author of 'Bonkers', Olivia's story of postnatal psychosis led her to start the Every Mum Movement, whose mission is to empower every mum to treat their mental health as importantly as their physical health.

everymummovement.com

Moodjuice

Fast and direct access to self-help resources for a range of mood disorders.

www.moodjuice.scot.nhs.uk

Positive Birth Movement

Author of the best-selling 'Positive Birth Book' Milli Hill founded the Positive Birth Movement which is a global network of free-to-access antenatal groups.

www.positivebirthmovement.org

Birthing Awareness Training

Birthing Awareness Training provides training and education around birth trauma and the birth debrief process, including training practitioners in the Rewind method.

www.birthingawarenesstraining.com

Birth Trauma Association

A charity that supports parents who suffer birth trauma.

www.birthtraumaassociation.org.uk

Anxiety UK

A charity supporting people suffering with anxiety.

www.anxietyuk.org.uk

WRAP®

The Wellness Action Recovery Plan® is a self-designed prevention and wellness process that anyone can use to get well, stay well and make their life the way they want it to be.

www.mentalhealthrecovery.com/wrap-is

Mind

The mental health charity.

www.mind.org.uk

Rethink Mental Illness

National mental health charity: information, services and a strong voice for anyone affected by mental illness.

www.rethink.org

National Institute of Mental Health

The world's largest scientific organisation dedicated to research focused on the understanding and treatment of mental illness.

www.nimh.nih.gov

Mental Health Foundation

Their mission is to help people understand, protect and sustain their mental health.

www.mentalhealth.org.uk

Time to Change

A growing movement of people changing how we think and act about mental health problems.

www.time-to-change.org.uk

PANDAS (Pre and Postnatal Depression Advice and Support)

Advice, support and links to local peer support groups in the UK including a helpline.

www.pandasfoundation.org.uk

Association for Postnatal Illness (APNI)

Support, education and information on postnatal mental illness.

www.apni.org

Postpartum Support International

Provides peer support, training to professionals and a bridge to connect them.

www.postpartum.net

Maternal Mental Health Alliance

A coalition of UK organisations with a vision to see all women across the UK get consistent, accessible and quality care and support for their mental health during pregnancy and in the year after giving birth.

www.maternalmentalhealthalliance.org

Headspace

An app which provides guided meditation on a range of themes such as anxiety, stress, insomnia and more.

www.headspace.com

Steps to Recovery

A resource for mental health recovery which gives personal accounts of people who have struggled with mental illness and the process they went through to recover.

www.mentalhealthrecoverystories.hscni.net

Centre for Clinical Interventions

A source of self-help worksheets for a range of disorders including depression, anxiety and obsessive-compulsive disorder.

www.cci.health.wa.gov.au/Resources/Looking-After-Yourself

Cry-sis

Offers support to families with excessively crying, sleepless and demanding babies.

www.cry-sis.org.uk

Mothers for Mothers

Postnatal depression support group and resource site.

www.mothersformothers.co.uk

MAMA: The 'Meet A Mum Association'

Self-help groups for mothers with small children.

www.mama.co.uk

Samaritans

Provides confidential, non-judgmental support 24 hours a day for people experiencing distress and despair, including those which could lead to suicide.

www.samaritans.org

Action on Postpartum Psychosis (APP)

A community for those affected by postnatal psychosis.

www.healthunlocked.com/app-network

Books

Lost Connections

By Johann Hari

Johann Hari uncovers the real cause of depression and anxiety and explores the unexpected solutions

Bonkers

By Olivia Siegl

A story of one woman's triumph over postnatal psychosis

Owning It: Your Bullshit-free Guide to Living with Anxiety

By Caroline Foran

An insightful and practical look into anxiety and what you can do to help yourself

The Body Keeps The Score

By Bessel Van Der Kolk

A look into how the body holds trauma and reflects the state of the brain and ways in which to help.

Men, Love and Birth

By Mark Harris

Mark explores how to harness the power of birthing hormones, how to remain calm and aware in the birthing room, how to communicate effectively and ultimately how to live the process of becoming a father to the full.

Daddy Blues: Postnatal Depression and Fatherhood

By Mark Williams

A touching story from a rarely explored perspective, this tells the tale of a man learning to deal with a postnatal depression.

Mindful Birthing: Training the Mind, Body and Heart for Birthing and Beyond

By Nancy Bardacke

Pioneering nurse-midwife Nancy Bardacke provides expectant families everywhere with the tools they need to reduce the stress, fear and pain associated with pregnancy and childbirth.

The Compassionate Mind Approach to Postnatal Depression

By Michelle Cree

Using compassion focused therapy to enhance mood, confidence and bonding

Fine (Not Fine): Perspectives and Experiences of Postnatal Depression

By Bridget Hargreave

Bridget Hargreave charts for own experiences of depression following the birth of her sons and records the histories of a collection of mothers with a diverse range of perinatal mental health problems.

Acknowledgements

This book is for my husband and children, and all the partners, children and families of those who are suffering with mental illness.

To my husband Eoin in particular, who has been my rock, my anchor, my rudder in what seemed to me a perilous and vast ocean of anxiety, depression and confusion. I couldn't have weathered these many storms without you. Thank you from the bottom of my heart for your patience, your love and your never-ending faith in me and for being the parent that our children needed when I couldn't be.

To my daddy. In the times where I felt numb and longed to feel some emotion, your sentimentality and memories of all our nights crying along to 'old' songs helped me to find the feelings again and bring them to the surface. Your humour and wit have often diffused an anxious moment and some of my fondest memories and experiences are those we shared, just the two of us. We have had our differences but you mean everything to me. I love you Papa Joe.

To my mummy. You have spent your life sacrificing for others, most of all your children. It is only now that I am a mother that I can appreciate the work and the exhaustion and the fear and the love you must have felt raising us. I wish I could go back in time and make life easier for you. I want you to have everything you deserve and I hope that you someday realise how incredible you are, and to begin to invest in your own wellbeing and happiness. I want you to know that I see you. And I love you.

To my sisters Angela and Nichola, and my baby brother Paul. It has been interesting being the odd one out among you. Sometimes I wish I was a bit more on the inside of the circle but mostly I love that despite our differences, we are all part of the same team. Thank you for all your support as I've worked through these difficult years: the messages, the phone calls, the company and the childcare! For trying to understand my struggle when I barely understood it myself and for listening to my endless self-analysis and not allowing me to wallow too long in my self-pity. While I hope that you never go through difficult days, I do hope that someday I can repay you for your love and support. I hope that you all know just how much I love you and want the very best for you.

To my mother- and father-in-law, Rosaleen and Eamon. You are the picture of kindness, generosity and loving care. You have welcomed me into your family so completely that I almost find the term 'in-law' offensive. You are as much a part of my family as my own and I thank you so fully from the bottom of my heart for bearing with me through those worrisome early days when the girl with bright pink hair threatened to corrupt your son! I hope to be as patient and accepting when my own children bring home partners of their own. Thank you also for being a listening ear when times have been rough and for never making me feel out of place. You have made not just our lives easier, but our marriage so much stronger for your support and guidance.

To my sisters from other misters: you know who you are! For joining me in my panic attacks, sharing my anxieties, helping me to untangle the complicated knot of mental illness, motherhood, womanhood and more! For recognising when I needed a friend and for always being at the end of the phone with commiseration, support, laughter and advice. In particular Tiarna and Gemma, who I have shared two of my maternity journeys with and who are the very essence of my tribe. You never failed to show up with tea and cake when I needed a friend. Those seemingly small acts were huge to me and made many difficult times that much more bearable.

To Michael, Glenna, Chad and Jennifer. Who would have thought that an school exchange trip could so completely transform a person's life? You showed a lost and confused girl the way to become a confident, fulfilled and enlightened woman. You continue to inspire me daily and when I am doubting myself and my abilities I think of you. Glenna, you are the woman I strive to be. Thank you all so much for the influence you have had in my life. Thank you for the love you give and the change you are creating in this world. I can only hope to be the role model for my children that you have been to me.

To the members of the PANGS NI support group. Wow. You have taken a simple idea, to find people who were like me, and you've transformed it into something beautiful. The support, care and love you show each other astounds me. You have seen me, and many others like me, through dark and difficult times. When I got lost on the road, you showed me the way. Your stories, your experiences and your knowledge have been the foundation on which PANGS is built and so many others are benefiting because of it. My hope is that you all find your peace and use your experience to guide others out of the darkness.

To Seána, Lindsay, Nuala and Catherine. We came together as five individuals wanting to make a difference and here we stand, a team, ready to take the fight where it needs to go in order to do better for our women. We all contribute in very different ways but this collaboration has changed me in ways you can't imagine. I look forward to long and fruitful relationships with you all and to sitting down one day to celebrate getting the services we are demanding. Keep striving, keep fighting. We will win.

To all my friends, too many to name. I am so grateful that chance brought you all into my life. We have grown up together and even when we go months without seeing each other, it is a comfort to know that we can pick up where we left off like no time had passed at all. We have dealt with our own challenges and I hope you all know that I think of you as family and my door is always open.

To Dave. You are a constant source of comfort, amusement and surprise. I love our debates, how we can chat for hours and never get bored. I love that you always make time to come to see me even when I have three little people hanging off my arms. I love that you take the time to engage with my children and never show your boredom when I go off on a birth-related tangent. Thank you.

To Mark and the team at Birthing Awareness. Thank you for believing in me. This book has been a birthing experience all of its own but one that you have handled with care and compassion. I am indebted to you for your support and willingness to take a chance on a difficult book and a complicated author. Thank you for allowing this book to shine a light on the otherwise shady topic of mental illness and for allowing me to do it on my own terms. You are amazing.

And finally, to my three children Alexis, Cooper and Luna. You made me the woman I am today. Having you changed my life in ways I could never imagine. Yes, there were dark times and worrying times and times when I wasn't the best mother I could be for you. But there were also joyous times and you have filled my heart so completely with love and adoration that it could explode! I hope you realise how deeply I love you and how I will spend the rest of my life loving you and doing whatever I can to help guide you through this funny thing called life. Perhaps when you look back at the times when I was less than perfect, you might realise I was doing my very best and that sometimes the mental illness just took over. I hope you know how often I kissed your head when you were sleeping and apologised to you, promising to do better the next day. I want you to know that you were my reason for fighting. For living. Wanting to be the best for you drove me forward in times when I felt like I couldn't even breathe. You are my life, my loves and I'm so proud to be your mother. I only hope you can be proud of me too. If you learn nothing else from me, learn this: be tenacious in your fight to have the best life. You will no doubt go through dark days of your own. When those days come, fight like hell to get back to the light because you are everything. You deserve everything. Surround yourselves with good friends, find yourselves partners who will love and support you no matter what. Most of all, know that you can always call on me. I love you all beyond words. You are the best thing I ever did.

Printed in Great Britain
by Amazon

54729172R00095